Asthma Management for Practice

D1766514

3310012800

WITHDRAWN
from
STIRLING UNIVERSITY LIBRARY

University of Stirling Library, FK9 4LA
Tel. 01786 – 467220

POPULAR LOAN

This Item is likely to be in heavy demand.
Please RETURN or RENEW no later
than the last date stamped below

- 6 APR 2001
- 3 MAY 2001
18 MAY 2001
10 JUL 2001
- 2 JUL 2001
- 9 JUL 2001
- 4 JUN 2002
14 JUN 2002

For Churchill Livingstone:

Commissioning editor: Alex Mathieson
Project manager: Valerie Burgess
Project editor: Valerie Dearing
Project controller: Derek Robertson
Design direction: Judith Wright
Copy editor: Colin Macnee
Indexer: Elizabeth Ball
Promotions manager: Hilary Brown

Asthma Management for Practice Nurses

A Psychological Perspective

Y
19E
HYL

Michael Hyland BSc PhD CPsychol
Professor of Health Psychology, Department of Psychology, Faculty of Human Science, University of Plymouth, UK

Foreword by

Greta Barnes MBE SRN
Director, National Asthma Respiratory Training Centre, Warwick, UK

POP

CHURCHILL
LIVINGSTONE

EDINBURGH LONDON NEW YORK PHILADELPHIA SAN FRANCISCO SYDNEY TORONTO 1998

74844
3/01

CHURCHILL LIVINGSTONE
A Division of Harcourt Brace and Company Limited
Churchill Livingstone, Robert Stevenson House, 1–3 Baxter's Place,
Leith Walk, Edinburgh EH1 3AF, UK

© Michael E Hyland 1998

is a registered trade mark of Harcourt Brace and Company Limited

All rights reserved. No part of this publication may by reproduced, stored in a retrieval system, or transmitted in any form or by any means, electronic, mechanical, photocopying, recording or otherwise, without either the prior permission of the publishers (Churchill Livingstone, Robert Stevenson House, 1–3 Baxter's Place, Leith Walk, Edinburgh EH1 3AF), or a licence permitting restricted copying in the United Kingdom issued by the Copyright Licensing Agency Ltd, 90 Tottenham Court Road, London, W1P 9HE.

The right(s) of Michael Hyland to be identified as author of this work has been asserted by him in accordance with the Copyright, Designs and Patent Act 1988.

First published 1998

ISBN 0 443 05682 X

British Library of Cataloguing in Publication Data
A catalogue record for this book is available from the British Library.

Library of Congress Cataloging in Publication Data
A catalog record for this book is available from the Library of Congress.

Medical knowledge is constantly changing. As new information becomes available, changes in treatment, procedures, equipment and the use of drugs become necessary. The author and the publishers have, as far as it is possible, taken care to ensure that the information given in this text is accurate and up-to-date. However, readers are strongly advised to confirm that information, especially with regard to drug usage, complies with the latest legislation and standards of practice.

The publisher's policy is to use **paper manufactured from sustainable forests**

Produced by Addison Wesley Longman China Limited, Hong Kong
EPC/01

Contents

Foreword

During the last 10 years the practice nurse has become a major provider of asthma care in the UK. Studies have shown that greater involvement by specially trained practice nurses in asthma management has been associated with improved outcomes.

Many nurses are now equipped to run an asthma clinic with autonomy. They provide a service which not only requires an ability to organise and manage but also requires teaching skills so patients can learn about the condition. Nurses give information about the various treatments, how they work, and how to choose (and use) an amazing array of inhaler devices, as well as how to manage an acute attack of asthma.

It is possible that the reason why these nurses are successful in improving care is because sufficient time is spent with the patient to allow scope not only to educate, but also to listen to the patient.

This book shows us, however, that there is much more to learn. It provides a valuable insight into the psychological management of patients who have asthma and shows how the nurse's role can be extended further.

There are excellent chapters on the effects of asthma on quality of life and compliance (or rather, 'non-compliance') issues. Also, very instructive sections on how to form a therapeutic relationship with patients, coping strategies and how to help patients manage their own asthma.

Michael Hyland is an acknowledged expert in the psychological aspects of asthma care and should be congratulated on producing a much-needed book for advanced practice nurses on how to understand patients and how to influence their behaviour.

G.B.
1998

About this book

There is a wide consensus that the majority of patients with asthma should be managed in primary care rather than secondary care. Many general practices have set up asthma clinics, often run by a practice nurse who is able to provide the time needed to educate patients about asthma management. This book is written with practice nurses in mind but will be of interest to any health professional who has a particular interest in the psychology of asthma management.

Three themes run through this book:

1. The pathophysiology and psychology of asthma are inextricably linked. One cannot be considered without the other. However, in many cases of poor asthma management, it is the psychological side which is causing the problem (e.g. the patient is not taking the drugs provided), rather than any inadequacy in the medicines themselves.
2. Patients differ both physiologically and psychologically and so need to be managed in different ways both from a physiological and a psychological perspective. The psychological differences are particularly important in asthma because many of the differences in outcome stem from psychological causes.
3. Patients have preferred methods of coping with asthma as well as having preferred type of quality of life, and both these preferences should be taken into account in asthma management.

The book starts with an introduction to the physiology of asthma (Ch. 1) (trained asthma nurses may find this chapter too superficial for their needs, and may wish to start the book at Ch. 2), moves on to the psychological consequences of asthma (Ch. 2), and then covers the initial physiological and psychological assessments (Ch. 3) which need to be taken in setting up a self-management plan. The book then links the psychology and physiology of asthma in terms of self-management plans (Chs 4 and 5) and compliance (Ch. 6), with a brief final chapter on organising an asthma clinic (Ch. 7).

Acknowledgements

This book would never have been started were it not for Greta Barnes. Nor would it have been finished were it not for the considerable help and kindness received from the many health professionals who have shared their experiences on asthma management with me over the years. There are too many to thank, but individuals may recognise a story they told me which I have used as an example or case study in the book. Finally, I am particularly grateful to Martyn Partridge for checking the book for physiological inaccuracies – but any errors are my own!

1 Introduction to physiological principles of asthma management

■ CONTENTS

WHAT IS ASTHMA?

Asthma is a disease causing *variable* obstruction of the airways, and the variability of airways obstruction is a defining feature of asthma. In this context, the word 'variable' means that the degree of obstruction varies over time for any one patient. However, the word 'variable' could also have another meaning, because the degree of the obstruction also varies between patients. Some patients have very

Box 1.1 Diagnostic definition of asthma

Asthma is defined as generalised narrowing of the airways, which varies over short periods of time either spontaneously or as a result of treatment.

mild asthma, and their management is different from those who have severe asthma. Successful management of asthma starts from these two basic facts: (a) asthma varies over short periods of time for any one patient, and (b) asthma varies in severity between patients. Consequently, (a) it may be necessary to change a patient's drugs from one occasion to another, and (b) different patients may be prescribed different drugs. Although this variability may give the impression that asthma management is complex, it is, in fact, relatively straightforward once the principles of disease process are understood. Four basic rules (listed below) underpin all asthma care.

There are two pathological processes causing airways obstruction: inflammation and bronchoconstriction. From the perspective of treatment, the inflammation is the more important because inflammation causes bronchoconstriction, but both inflammation and bronchoconstriction can be treated by drug therapy.

Inflammation

Asthma is a type of autoimmune disease, because the body's own defence system is responsible for the inflammation. White blood cells in the lung attack the lining of the airways, releasing chemicals which encourage further attack. The attacking white blood cells (several different types are involved) cause a reddening of the inside of the airways. At the same time, the damaged inside walls begin puffing up, and this narrows the tube. The damaged tube linings also start producing a lot of mucus which flows around the inside of the tubes, and the excessive mucus also narrows the tube. Mucus is normally swept up the airways and out into the mouth by the cilia lining the inside of the airways, which beat upwards. However, where there is excessive mucus, or where there is a lot of damage to the inside of the walls of the airways, these little hairs do not work effectively. As a result the mucus tends to accumulate in the form of plugs which can block up a tube completely. In short, inflammation causes an obstruction for one reason or another, and the obstruction leads to asthma symptoms and the risk of asthma attack (Fig. 1.1).

Inflammation is due to overactivity of white blood cells, and all anti-inflammatory drugs work one way or another by reducing the activity of these white blood cells – either by inhibiting them directly or by interfering with the chemicals that stimulate white blood cell activity. The more the white blood cells cause inflammation, the greater is the need for anti-inflammatory medication. Amongst the population of asthma patients, the degree of inflammation caused by the white blood cells varies. Without treatment, the level of inflammation varies from the very severe to the very mild, and the mild merges imperceptibly with the normal lung. Consequently the strength of anti-inflammatory medicine needed will also vary.

- ***Rule 1***: *The strength of anti-inflammatory medication needed depends on the degree to which the patient's white blood cells cause inflammation.*

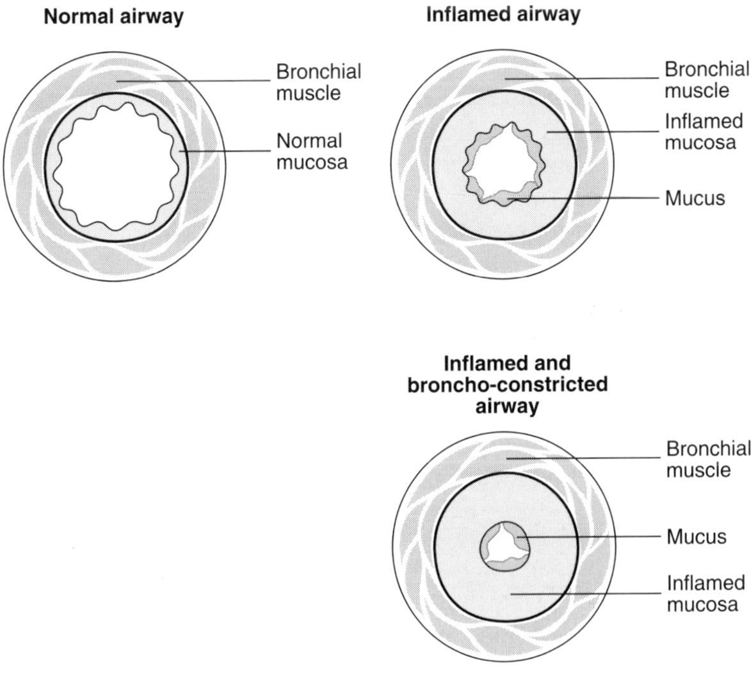

Fig. 1.1 Causes of airways obstruction in asthma.

The inflammatory action of the white blood cells is increased by environmental factors, and is also subject to intrinsic variation for reasons which are not well understood. Because of this, the need for anti-inflammatory medication varies over time. One possible way of dealing with this variation is to ensure that the patient has sufficiently strong anti-inflammatory medication to cover normal day-to-day variation in inflammation, but to make provision for increased anti-inflammatory medication when needed.

- ***Rule** 2: There may be occasions when the normally prescribed anti-inflammatory medicine is insufficient, and an increase in dose becomes necessary.*

Bronchoconstriction

The smooth muscles of the airways are capable of contracting in a person without asthma, and they do so when the airways become irritated, for example by smoke. However, the nonasthmatic airways do not contract very much. In the patient with asthma, however, the airways have an enhanced capacity for bronchoconstriction from irritation. The airways are 'twitchy' in the sense that they constrict easily when triggered by circumstances which have little or no effect on people who do not have asthma, and they also contract to a greater extent. This twitchyness of the airways is called bronchial hyper-responsiveness.

The main reason for bronchial hyper-responsiveness is inflammation. Simply put, inflammation causes twitchiness, and it is for this reason that anti-inflammatory medicines are crucial to asthma control. However, the bronchial hyper-responsiveness is only noticed in the presence of a trigger – in the absence of a trigger the hyper-responsive airways do not constrict (Fig. 1.2).

Bronchodilating medicines stimulate receptors (β receptors) in the airways muscles, causing them to relax. There are several reasons why bronchodilating medicines are prescribed.

1. The asthma may be so mild and symptoms occur so infrequently that occasional use of bronchodilators is sufficient. The patient therefore keeps a bronchodilator (normally a β-agonist stimulant) available for use when needed.
2. Although symptoms are usually controlled by anti-inflammatory medicine (normally an inhaled steroid), occasionally

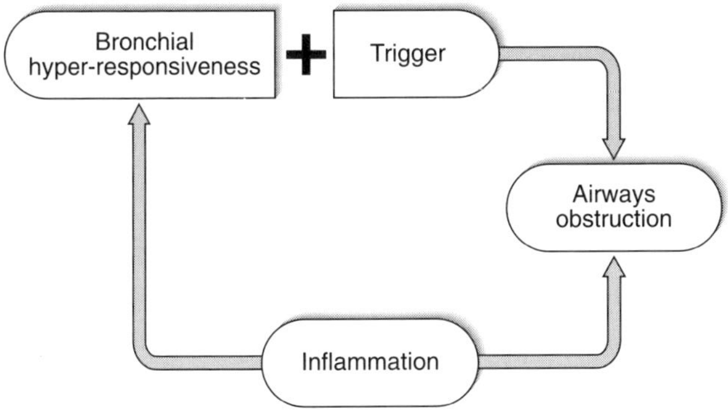

Fig. 1.2 Causal relationships in asthma.

bronchoconstriction occurs, either because it is triggered by something in the environment or because of intrinsic variability, and so there is a need for bronchodilators as well. The patient therefore keeps a bronchodilator available for use when needed.

3. Adequate control of asthma symptoms in some cases can only be achieved by constant application of both anti-inflammatory and bronchodilating medicine. The patient therefore uses bronchodilators daily.

- ***Rule 3***: *Bronchodilators should be used, irregularly or regularly, only when insufficient control of asthma is achieved through anti-inflammatory medicine.*

It is important to emphasise that control of inflammation is the major objective of asthma management, and that anti-inflammatory and bronchodilating medicines should be used in very different ways.

It follows from Rules 2 and 3 that there will need to be *variation* in the way both anti-inflammatory and bronchodilating medicines are taken. This variation requires the patient to follow a self-management plan. The patient has to know how to alter the medicines taken on a day-to-day basis, and to know when to get help from a health professional.

- ***Rule 4***: *Effective asthma management requires the patient to be actively involved in managing his or her asthma.*

Active involvement of the patient places an extra responsibility on the health professional. Asthma care is not simply a matter of giving patients prescriptions. Asthma care also involves teaching and motivating patients to manage their own asthma in an effective and safe way.

Objective measurement of obstruction and peak expiratory flow

Objective measurement of airways obstruction is possible because the obstruction alters airflow. Breathing out is a passive process where the muscles which expand the rib cage and the muscles of the diaphragm relax, and in so doing the alveoli push air out through the bronchioles and bronchi, rather like letting down millions of tiny balloons (about 250 million balloons altogether). The rate with which these tiny balloons can be let down is determined by the degree of airways obstruction, rather in the same way that the rate with which a balloon expels air is reduced if an obstruction is placed in the outlet. The maximum rate at which air can be expelled by the lungs is therefore a measure of airways obstruction, assuming, of course, that the muscles controlling inspiration are relaxed suddenly.

There are several ways in which the rate of air expelled from the lungs can be measured. One way is to measure the amount of air expelled during the first second of blowing — which is called forced expiratory volume in the first second, or FEV_1. In a person without lung disease, the total capacity of the lung, or forced vital capacity (FVC), is expelled in just slightly more than 1 s, but the person with asthma has a much reduced rate of expiration (Fig. 1.3).

FEV_1 is probably the most accurate way of measuring obstruction, but it requires a spirometer, which is a comparatively expensive piece of equipment. Although available in hospitals, spirometers are often not available in the asthma clinic – though the introduction of 'mini' spirometers means that some primary care clinics purchase them. An alternative method, and one which is very nearly as good, is to measure peak expiratory flow rate, or PEF. PEF is a measure of the fastest rate that air can be expelled from the lungs, and the equipment needed to measure it is called a peak flow meter. Peak flow meters, and in particular 'mini wright' peak flow meters, are very cheap – cheap enough to provide to patients on the NHS so that they can measure their own PEF.

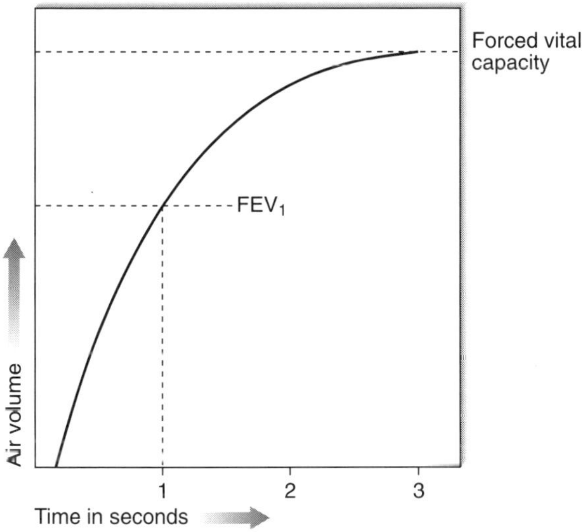

Fig. 1.3 Rate at which air is expelled from the lungs in a person with asthma.

Airways obstruction is variable over time, and so is PEF. The advantage of giving patients their own peak flow meter is that they can measure the obstruction over time, and this advantage substantially outweighs the greater accuracy of spirometry. Hence, in primary care, the peak flow meter is the standard therapeutic tool for measuring airways obstruction. By contrast, the spirometer is more useful as a diagnostic tool: not only is it more accurate, but the relationship between FEV_1 and FVC is a useful diagnostic indicator.

When using a peak flow meter, the patient stands upright, takes a deep breath, puts the lips firmly round the mouthpiece and blows out as hard as possible. The patient's PEF rate can be read off on a scale in litres per minute, taking the best of three blows to reduce measurement error. A high PEF indicates good lung function, and a low PEF poor lung function, where 'lung function' is used as a general term to describe how effective the lungs are. The PEF value can be compared with the predicted value for a person who is nonasthmatic. As the predicted value for PEF varies with age and height as well as gender, it is necessary to look up the predicted value from tables or from a figure. Figure 1.4 provides information on PEF in normal (i.e., nonasthmatic) adults in a way which permits easy comparison with individual patients.

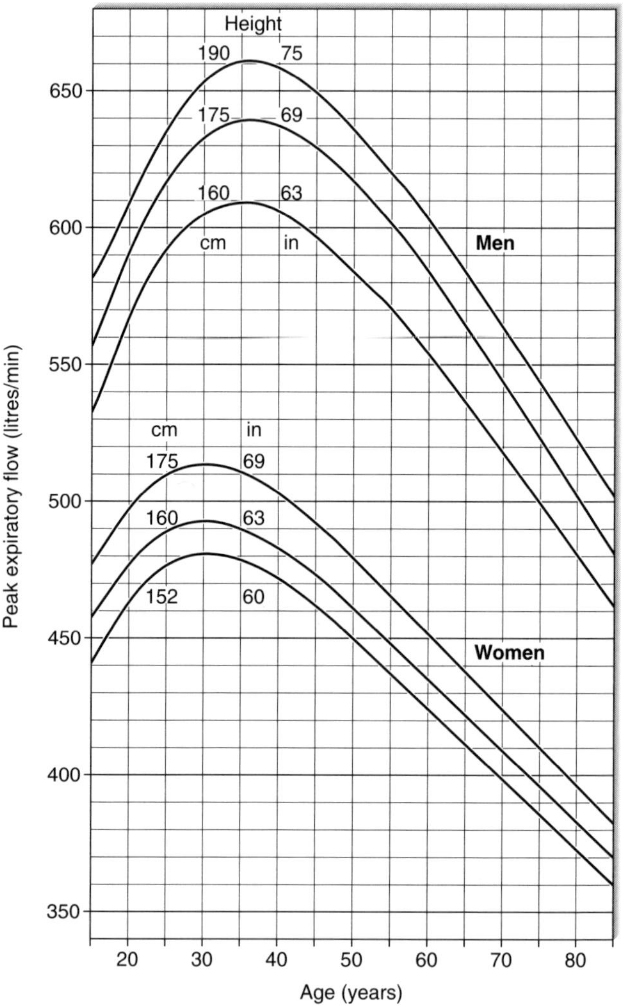

Fig. 1.4 Peak expiratory flow rate in normal adults. From Gregg and Nunn (1989).

In people without asthma, lung function varies slightly over the course of the day. In the morning it is slightly lower than in the evening. In the poorly controlled asthma patient, the morning/evening variation is very much greater, and in addition the average value of PEF tends to be lower. The relationship between daily PEF variation in people with and without asthma is shown in Figure 1.5

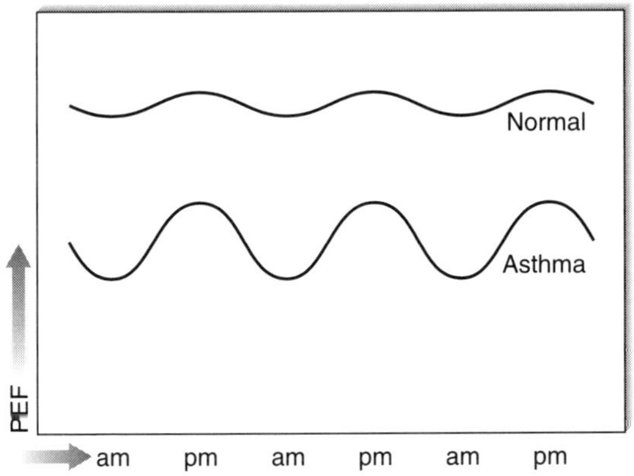

Fig. 1.5 Variation in peak expiratory flow rate for people with and without asthma.

The pattern of PEF change shown in Figure 1.5 is a kind of theoretical representation of changes that occur. The reality tends to be rather different, as the pattern of change in patients with asthma is much more random, reflecting a variety of intrinsic and extrinsic factors affecting lung function. In practice, a PEF graph tends to look rather messy, and an example is shown in Figure 1.6

Measurement of PEF is useful for health professionals because it provides information about the severity of disease, what may be triggering it, and the effectiveness of treatment. Hence, knowledge of

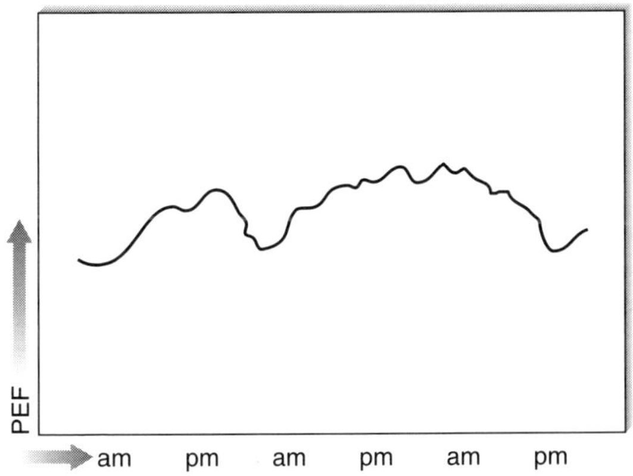

Fig. 1.6 Example of a PEF graph.

PEF is particularly important for deciding the level of medication required. Values of PEF lower than 80% predicted, or where there is diurnal variation of more than 15%, would be indicative of pathology. Of course, the patient may be on effective medication, in which case PEF will appear more similar or indeed identical to normal lung function.

Diagnosis and types of asthma

Asthma can be diagnosed by its reversible nature using the objective measurement of lung function provided by PEF. Evidence for asthma is provided by any one of the following.

- Variation of PEF is greater than 15% over any time period.
- PEF falls by more than 15% after exercise. PEF should be measured and then again after about 5 min of exercise (Fig. 1.7).
- PEF improves by more than 15% after inhaling a bronchodilating drug.

The value of 15% in the above criteria is a convention, nothing more than that. The reality is that asthma merges imperceptibly with the normal, and 15% is the level at which most people think it reasonable to classify someone as having asthma. Of course, there will be people who are 15% reversible perhaps one or two occasions in the year, or just at particular seasons of the year. Classification of asthma at these low levels is a matter of judgement.

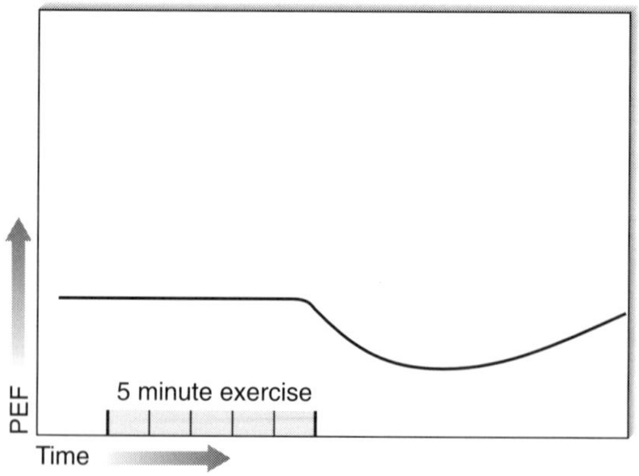

Fig. 1.7 Decrease in PEF following exercise in poorly controlled asthma.

Diagnosis of asthma is normally carried out by the GP and difficult cases of diagnosis referred to a respiratory consultant (see Ch. 6), who will carry out additional tests. Low PEF is indicative of asthma but not diagnostic, because other lung diseases also have low PEF. Similarly, the presence of symptoms is indicative but not diagnostic of asthma. Some other lung diseases are shown in Table 1.1.

There are several types of asthma, reflecting different types of inflammatory processes, though differences between these types are not well understood. It is common to distinguish between atopic (or allergic) and nonatopic (or nonallergic) asthma. Atopic asthma runs in families, has a genetic predisposition in common with eczema and rhinitis, and tends to appear early – i.e., in childhood (also called early-onset asthma). Nonatopic asthma does not run in families and tends to onset later in life (also called late-onset asthma). The presence of asthma in the family, and to a slightly lesser extent eczema and rhinitis, makes asthma more likely. Therefore presence of familial asthma, eczema and rhinitis indicates a possibility of asthma if patients are symptomatic. Although atopic and nonatopic asthma may be triggered by different environmental features (see later), the difference between these types is otherwise not important in terms of patient management.

There are reports of underdiagnosis of asthma in elderly people. Although there is a peak of asthma incidence in childhood (about 5

Table 1.1 Some other lung diseases

Airways diseases	**Restrictive disorders**	**Other causes of breathlessness**
Localised	*Lung diseases*	Hyperventilation
Carcinomas	Sarcoidosis	Anxiety
Foreign bodies	Asbestosis	Vascular diseases
Vocal cord paresis	Fibrosing alveolitis	Infection
Generalised	*Pleural diseases*	
Asthma	Effusions	
Chronic obstructive pulmonary disease	Pneumothorax	
Cystic fibrosis		
Obliterative bronchiolitis		

Note: diagnosis requires specialist opinion.

years) which then declines, asthma incidence starts increasing again after about 40 or 50 years. Asthma may develop for the first time in elderly people. The reason for the underdiagnosis is uncertain, but elderly people may confuse their symptoms with that of growing old and therefore not report for diagnosis. In addition, elderly people tend to perceive a given level of airways narrowing less readily than younger people. Also, asthma in elderly people shares symptoms with chronic obstructive pulmonary disease (COPD), a nonreversible airways disease which occurs in older people, and typically with smokers. However, elderly smokers can develop a mixture of asthma and COPD, and may attribute their symptoms to smoking rather than to either disease. Whatever the reason for this underdiagnosis, it indicates the need to be aware of wheeze or breathlessness in elderly patients even when patients do not complain about their breathing.

DOES HAVING ASTHMA MATTER?

Prevalence and aims of management

Asthma affects about 4–5% of the adult population, and drug costs alone in 1993 were £350 million. Although it is rare, asthma can cause death – there are about one and a half thousand deaths per year in the UK in a population of nearly three million asthma patients. Asthma deaths in UK people under 65 fell considerably between 1986 and 1992 (Department of Health 1994). Despite this improvement, it is widely believed that more asthma deaths could be avoided through more effective management. In addition to the risk of death, asthma detracts from quality of life. Impairment of quality of life is a much more common consequence of asthma than is death. Asthma matters because, if it is poorly managed, it can lead to death, and because, even with good management, it can have an impact, sometimes a substantial impact, on quality of life.

The three fundamental aims of asthma management are:

- to reduce the risk of asthma death
- to improve the quality of life of the patient, both in the present and for the future
- to reduce the risk of airways narrowing becoming fixed and irreversible.

In addition, and because of budgetary constraints, some practices add an additional aim (discussed in Ch. 7):

- to achieve the above aims in a cost-effective manner.

Airways obstruction and activity

Lungs have the function of delivering oxygen into the blood stream, and in the normal person they have plenty of spare capacity. When a person engages in maximal physical effort (for example, when running) then it is the skeletal muscles (for example, the leg muscles) that limit physical ability. Physical activity is not normally restricted by the limitations imposed by the lungs. Because lungs do not normally limit activity, most people are unaware of their breathing. However, when lung function is poor, then it is the lungs rather than the skeletal muscles that limit activity. Thus, the person with asthma experiences a kind of limitation when running – sometimes even when walking – that is not experienced by other people: namely physical limitation due to oxygen depletion. Activities are limited by the lungs, not by the skeletal muscles.

Asthma attacks

PEF varies between people and for any person with asthma over time. If PEF drops very substantially – for example, less than 150 L/min – then the patient may develop an asthma attack. An asthma attack occurs when the patient becomes distressed by asthma symptoms due to the low PEF and the symptoms are not readily relieved by a bronchodilating medicine. There are several reasons why the bronchodilator may be ineffective on a particular occasion, but a common one is that inflammation has developed without the patient's being aware or taking remedial action. An asthma attack is very dangerous, as lung function can gradually decline, leading to death from oxygen starvation. Patients are advised as part of their self-management plan to seek medical assistance in the case of asthma attacks (i.e., symptoms which do not respond to normal self-management), and such patients require *acute asthma treatment*. This book deals with *chronic asthma management*, where the aim is to prevent asthma attacks. Nevertheless, health professionals who provide chronic asthma management should familiarise themselves with the general principles of acute asthma treatment, and guidelines for acute attacks are provided in the British Thoracic Society's

Box 1.2 Asthma attack – degrees of severity

The phrase 'asthma attack' is not very precise, and both patients and health professionals use it in different ways. In practice there is a continuum between bronchospasm where the patient will get better only after acute treatment by a health professional (either at the patient's home, in the clinic, or in hospital), bronchospasm where the patient will get better gradually following self-treatment and time to sit down, relax and recover, and bronchospasm which is relieved relatively quickly by a bronchodilator.

general guidelines on asthma (British Thoracic Society 1990, 1993, British Asthma Guidelines Coordinating Committee 1997). Asthma attacks are rare, but their serious consequences mean that they are an important consideration in asthma management.

Asthma symptoms

People with asthma report symptoms. The symptoms can coincide with decreases in PEF, but the relationship between PEF and symptoms is often poor (see later). The four main symptoms of asthma are:

- *breathlessness* – awareness of breathing; a feeling of difficulty or work when breathing; a feeling of being out of breath; a feeling of being unable to expel air from the chest (sometimes called by patients 'puffiness')
- *chest tightness* – a feeling of heaviness or weight on the chest
- *wheeze* – a breathing sound which is audible to the patient, and to other people standing close by
- *cough* – a cough which can be no different from coughs having other causes.

Patients vary in the way they experience asthma symptoms: for example, some will notice the cough most of all whereas others may report no cough but are troubled by breathlessness. Patients can experience symptoms at any time in the day or night. Day-time symptoms can, but do not necessarily, affect the patient's quality of life. Night-time symptoms often wake the patient.

The asthma symptoms do not allow a diagnosis of asthma, but they indicate the need for asthma tests (see above). Chest tightness

Box 1.3 Example

The sensation of asthmatic breathlessness can be mimicked in nonasthmatic people. First, concentrate on breathing in and out normally. Notice that the breathing is quite shallow, and that it occurs with the lungs in an uninflated condition – i.e., when the lungs are mainly empty of air. Second, take a deep breath, so that the airways are at least 50% inflated, and continue with your previous shallow breathing but with a hyperinflated chest. Notice how it requires more effort to breathe in and out with a hyperinflated chest. Third, purse your lips and breathe in and out of your mouth allowing you lips to create an obstruction on the airflow. Notice how this makes matters worse. If you continue with obstructed breathing for a while, you will start getting tired which is one of the symptoms of an asthma attack.

and wheeze are characteristic symptoms of asthma but may also be found in patients with other respiratory diseases (e.g., obstructive pulmonary disease, emphysema, sarcoidosis, lung cancer). Cough is found in both people with asthma and people with and without other lung diseases. Breathlessness may arise simply by breathing too much air (hyperventilation). A simple test of hyperventilation is to ask the patient to take several deep breaths. If taking deep breaths increases symptoms (such as giddiness) then the patient may be a hyperventilator rather than having asthma.

ASTHMA TRIGGERS

An asthma trigger is anything that causes bronchoconstriction. Asthma triggers usually have a relatively rapid effect causing bronchoconstriction to occur fairly rapidly, i.e., in a matter of seconds or minutes. The particular triggers that cause bronchoconstriction vary between patients but they fall into six categories.

Small airborne particles and allergic reactions

Any airborne particle in 'dirty air' tends to irritate the lining of the airways when breathed; the very small airborne particles are particularly irritating to lung tissue. There are many types of airborne particles, and they include traffic fumes, cigarette smoke, air freshener, polishes, perfume, pollen, fungal spores, as well as the dander (small flakes of skin) which come off animals, particularly cats. One particularly important type of irritant is the faeces of house dust mites which live in carpets and household furnishings.

Sometimes patients develop an allergic reaction to airborne particles, particularly if the particles contain protein. The dander from cats, dogs and horses can sometimes produce this allergic reaction, and when an allergic reaction is involved, then the bronchoconstriction can be very much more rapid and intense. Other common triggers causing allergic reactions include house dust mite, and pollens and fungal spores. Seasonal asthma, for example, when the patient develops asthma only in the spring or only in the autumn is often due to allergic reactions to pollen and fungi, respectively. Allergic bronchoconstriction tends to be more severe than the irritant effect of small particles. As there is an allergic component in atopic asthma, patients tend to respond differently to different kinds of 'dirty air'. Dirty air which contains particles capable of creating an allergic reaction has a more bronchoconstricting effect than just plain dirty air. However, the particles which cause an allergic reaction differ substantially between patients.

Airborne gases and weather

Several gases irritate the airways. Sulphur dioxide, which is produced by some industrial processes, is particularly important in this respect, but other gases produced by photochemical processes in the air, such as ozone, can also have an effect. Because of the effect of weather on gases, as well as on airborne particles, weather conditions can have a substantial effect on asthma – as indicated, for example, by the relationship between the weather and frequency of emergency admissions.

Exercise and rapid breathing

Exercise leads to a more rapid flow of air through the airways, and the rapid airflow can act as a bronchoconstrictor. The way exercise affects patients varies a lot. For some, it is only cold air that is detrimental, and exercise inside a heated building leads to no problems. For others it is dry air which is detrimental, so that exercise in a swimming pool leads to no problems. On the other hand, some patients are irritated by the chlorine in swimming pools (i.e., the effect of a gas in the air). For some patients, rapid breathing brought about by laughter can have a bronchoconstricting effect.

Colds and other viral infections

Colds and other viral infections are very common asthma triggers. Some patients develop asthma symptoms even before they notice the symptoms of a cold. Some patients only develop asthma symptoms when they have a cold. Patients who are sensitive to colds often experience colds more badly because the infection then seems to go to the chest.

Psychological factors

A large number of patients develop bronchoconstriction from psychological factors. The most common psychological bronchoconstrictor is stress; in particular the stress associated with interpersonal conflict seems to be particularly harmful. Asthma attacks occur not infrequently after the patients have had a row. However, other forms of stress, for example anxiety over performance, can also lead to bronchoconstriction.

A second, less common psychological factor affecting lung function is expectancy. The expectation that bronchoconstriction will occur acts, for some patients, as a self-fulfilling prophecy. The expectancy need not be conscious. Some patients who are allergic to cats develop bronchoconstriction when they look at a picture of a cat, and a substantial number of patients exhibit bronchodilation when breathing in a placebo bronchodilator. Some patients develop symptoms if they realise that they have gone out without taking their bronchodilating medicine with them.

Food sensitivity

Food can act as a trigger in a minority of patients. There are two types of reaction to food: an immediate reaction where PEF starts to drop about 20–30 min after eating food (but can drop immediately), and a late reaction which occurs much more gradually, and is therefore more difficult to detect.

Hormones and drugs

Some women have a premenstrual decline in PEF. Some drugs can act as a trigger, in particular nonsteroidal anti-inflammatory agents (including aspirin and ibuprofen), as well as beta-blockers both as tablets and eye drops.

General features of triggers

The triggers which cause bronchoconstriction vary substantially between patients: some would have triggers from all categories above, some from only one. When levels of inflammation are high then triggers tend to produce a greater degree of constriction, and, because of intrinsic variation in inflammation, there is also intrinsic variability in sensitivity to some triggers. Thus, the extent to which a trigger actually triggers bronchoconstriction varies to some extent over time.

Some triggers, and particularly allergic triggers, can exacerbate inflammation. Therefore, for some triggers there is a short-term bronchoconstricting effect as well as a longer-term inflammatory effect. It goes without saying that there is less morbidity when the patient avoids triggers.

TREATING ASTHMA

Cure versus treatment

Asthma is not cured by asthma medicines. Asthma medicines control the pathological processes (inflammation and bronchodilation) but do not abolish them. Asthma medicines, both anti-inflammatories and bronchodilators, are normally taken by inhalation, with a few exceptions where the route of administration is oral. The reason for inhaled delivery of drugs is that the drug is delivered directly to the site where it is needed, thereby reducing side effects from systemic use.

What are asthma guidelines?

Asthma guidelines provide information about which drugs to prescribe, and advice about other aspects of management. They are guidelines, not rules, and provide scope for alternative strategies to be taken in individual cases. Several asthma guidelines have been published by societies associated with asthma care, both in the UK and abroad. The reason why it was felt necessary to publish guidelines was that asthma care can be variable in quality – i.e., different health care professionals did different things. To put it bluntly, some patients receive better care than others (Griffiths et al 1997). Asthma guidelines have had a major impact in improving both the consistency and quality of care provided.

The most commonly used guidelines in the UK are the 'British Thoracic Society Guidelines' or BTS guidelines. In fact a variety of other bodies also contributed to these guidelines, including patient groups, so they are actually representative of a variety of opinion, though the label reflects the fact that the British Thoracic Society was the driving force in their creation. First published in 1990, they were republished in 1993 with a 'revision' published in 1997, and the comparatively small changes between these different versions reflect changes in available medicines and management policies (British Thoracic Society 1990, 1993, British Asthma Guidelines Coordinating Committee 1997). The guidelines are based on a mixture of clinical experience and research findings, and are specifically designed to be 'user friendly' to health professionals. The BTS guidelines are particularly recommended for health professionals wanting a good practical set of instructions on how to manage asthma.

Although drawing on evidence, the BTS guidelines do not provide an evaluation of the evidence for the various recommendations, and they are therefore not strictly speaking evidence-based guidelines. Evidence-based guidelines were published by the North of England Asthma Guideline Development Group in 1996, and these evaluate the evidence for the different recommendations associated with asthma care. The North of England guidelines are particularly recommended for health professionals with an interest in research or who want to find out the evidence supporting management for patients.

The International Consensus Report on Diagnosis and Treatment of Asthma was published in 1992, and is a set of guidelines developed in the USA in conjunction with other countries. The international consensus report has been particularly influential in the USA.

Although the UK and international guidelines are very similar, there are differences in the way asthma is managed internationally. Broadly speaking, in the UK and in the rest of Europe there is a tendency to treat inflammation even in comparatively mild asthmatic patients with inhaled steroids – a practice consistent with the guidelines. In Japan and in the USA, inhaled steroids have in the past been introduced at a slightly later stage and in a lower dose – though the constant development of new drugs means that comparisons between countries can change. The reason for the early introduction of steroids in the UK and Europe is growing evidence that uncontrolled inflammation may have long-term adverse effects – i.e., compromise the patient's quality of life in older age.

The British Thoracic Society guidelines

The British Thoracic Society (BTS) guidelines are widely respected internationally; they are well written and easy to follow. The following should be considered as an overview and not a replacement for a document which is essential reading for those involved in asthma care.

The principle of treatment steps

The basic principle underlying the BTS guidelines is to divide treatment into five steps, each of which involves a gradual increase in the potency of asthma medicines prescribed. If asthma is not controlled at a lower step, then one moves up to the next step in the sequence. The aim is to position the patient on the lowest step that controls that patient's asthma. There has been one main change between the 1993 guidelines and the 1997 revision. When an uncontrolled patient presents in the clinic, the earlier guidelines (i.e., 1993 and before) suggested that one should step up until reaching control. The more recent guidelines (1997) suggest that one should go in at a higher level, establish control, and then step down. However, the end result is the same: the patient's physiological morbidity is counteracted by the use of drugs, but using the minimum amount of drug needed to achieve control.

The five steps of asthma management are based on the principle of gradually increasing treatment, and the steps plus commentary are shown in Table 1.2. The drugs themselves will be introduced in a later section.

If asthma is poorly controlled in terms of symptoms, PEF or activity restriction, then the management guidelines suggest that the treatment step should be increased. However, some patients have such severe asthma that even at Step 4 or Step 5 their asthma is not properly controlled, and so at Steps 4 and 5 the aim is to achieve the best possible control of asthma.

Table 1.2 British Thoracic Society treatment steps and commentary

BTS step as described in 1997 guidelines	**Commentary**
Step 1 Occasional use of relief bronchodilators Inhaled, short-acting β-agonists 'as required' for symptom relief are acceptable. If they are needed more than once daily, move to Step 2. Before altering a treatment step, ensure that the patient is having the treatment and has a good inhaler technique. Address any fears	Short-acting bronchodilators are prescribed to be used by the patient only when needed – i.e., when symptomatic
Step 2 Regular inhaled anti-inflammatory agents Inhaled, short-acting β-agonists as required, *plus* beclomethasone or budesonide 100–400 μg twice daily or fluticasone 40–200 μg twice daily; alternatively, use sodium cromoglycate or nedocromil sodium, but, if control is not achieved, start inhaled steroids	Regular mild/moderate anti-inflammatory drugs, plus short-acting bronchodilators when needed
Step 3 High-dose inhaled steroids or low-dose inhaled steroids plus long-acting β-agonist bronchodilator Inhaled, short-acting β-agonists as required, *plus either* beclomethasone or budesonide increased to 800–2000 μg daily or fluticasone 400–1000 μg daily via a large-volume spacer *or* beclomethasone or budesonide 100–400 μg twice daily or fluticasone 50–200 μg twice daily plus salmeterol 50 μg twice daily.	*Either* regular strong anti-inflammatory drugs, plus short-acting bronchodilators when needed *or* regular mild/moderate anti-inflammatory drugs, plus regular long-acting bronchodilators, plus short-acting bronchodilators when needed Note: further comment on this option in treatment is contained in Chapter 5

Table 1.2 *Cont'd*

BTS step as described in 1997 guidelines	Commentary
In a very small number of patients who experience side effects with high-dose inhaled steroids, either the long-acting inhaled β-agonist option is used or a sustained-release theophylline may be added to Step 2 medication. Cromoglycate or nedocromil may also be tried.	
Step 4 High-dose inhaled steroids and regular bronchodilators Inhaled short-acting β-agonists as required, with inhaled beclomethasone or budesonide 800–2000 μg daily via a large volume spacer, *plus* a sequential therapeutic trial of one or more of the following: – inhaled long-acting β-agonists – sustained release theophylline – inhaled ipratropium or oxitropium – long-acting β-agonist tablets – high-dose inhaled bronchodilators – cromoglycate or nedocromil	Regular strong anti-inflammatory drugs, plus regular long-acting bronchodilators, plus short-acting bronchodilators when needed
Step 5 Addition of regular steroid tablets Inhaled short-acting β-agonists as required, with inhaled beclomethasone or budesonide 800–2000 μg daily or fluticasone 400–1000 μg daily via a large-volume spacer, and one or more of the long-acting bronchodilators, *plus* regular prednisolone tablets in a single daily dose	Regular strong anti-inflammatory drugs, plus regular long-acting bronchodilators, plus regular oral steroids, plus short-acting bronchodilators when needed

Progression and ceiling dose

The progression through the steps depends on the degree of inflammation. The more inflammation, the greater the need for anti-inflammatory medicine. But there is a limit to the efficacy of any anti-inflammatory medicine. What seems to happen is that the anti-inflammatory effect of any anti-inflammatory medicine increases up to a particular level when a 'ceiling effect' is achieved. The ceiling dose is the dose at which further increase in dosage has no (or little) effect (Fig. 1.8). The ceiling dose varies with the patient, but the exact level and variation are not well understood. It is generally thought that the ceiling dose occurs in the region of 1000–2000 μg daily of beclomethasone via metered dose inhaler (MDI) or equivalent, but for some patients it may be well below that level (Kamada et al 1996).

For some patients the ceiling dose of a particular drug is enough or more than enough to control the patient's inflammation, so the patient only needs to be managed by that particular anti-inflammatory medicine. In other cases, the ceiling dose of the particular anti-inflammatory agent does not actually completely control the asthma. Two options then become available. One option is to add a long-acting bronchodilator as part of regular therapy. Thus, the addition of long-acting bronchodilators comes in at Step 3 or greater. Notice how at Step 3 there are two alternatives: (a) strong anti-inflammatories or (b) mild/moderate anti-inflammatories plus long-acting β-agonists. The reason for this alternative stems from differences between patients in the ceiling dose. Because the ceiling dose varies between patients, some patients benefit from earlier introduction of long-acting bronchodilators compared with others. Consequently, regular long-acting bronchodilators are added either

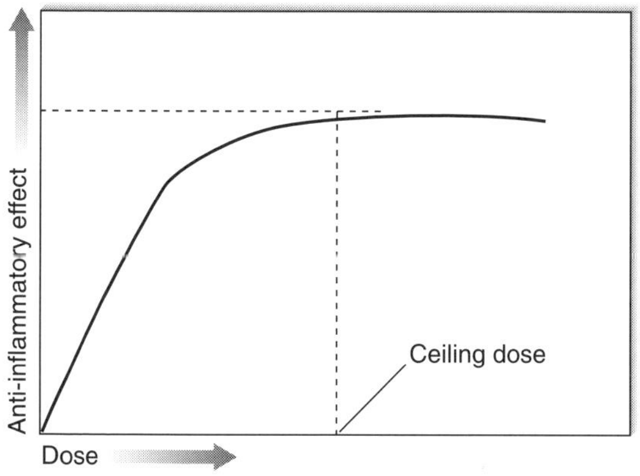

Fig. 1.8 Ceiling effect on efficacy of anti-inflammatory medicine.

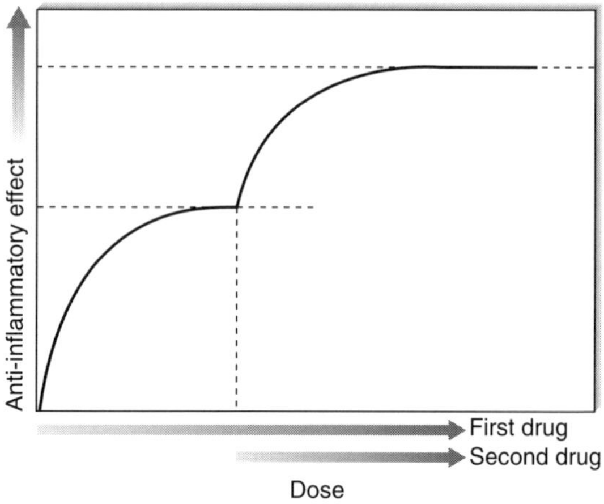

Fig. 1.9 Additive effect of two different anti-inflammatory drugs.

at Step 3 or Step 4, depending on the patient's response, which in itself depends on differences in physiology between patients.

When the ceiling dose of an anti-inflammatory drug is achieved, a second option is to add another type of anti-inflammatory drug of a different drug type. Two different anti-inflammatories which work in different ways can have an additive effect (Fig. 1.9). That is, together the two drugs push the anti-inflammatory ceiling higher. The consequence of the additive effect of anti-inflammatories is that a strong anti-inflammatory effect may be achievable through the use of two mild/moderate anti-inflammatories; or that a strong effect can be made even stronger by adding extra anti-inflammatory medicines of a different type to the current one. The combination of different types of anti-inflammatories is important at higher steps in the BTS guidelines (Steps 4 and 5) but may become more important at lower steps in the future with the development of new anti-inflammatory medicines.

TYPES OF MEDICINES

Anti-inflammatories

Anti-inflammatory drugs are of two classes: steroidal and nonsteroidal. Within each of these classes there are several different types of drug available.

Steroids

There are three different drugs used in the UK as inhaled steroids, and these are (in order of discovery):

- beclomethasone
- budesonide
- fluticasone.

Beclomethasone and budesonide are equally efficacious at similar dose, but fluticasone is twice as efficacious at a similar dose to the other two drugs. In practical terms, this means that the same level of anti-inflammatory effect can be achieved with fluticasone at half the dose. The side effect profiles of the three drugs are not identical, but see Chapter 5.

There is one commonly used oral steroid:

- prednisolone.

Nonsteroids

At the time of writing, two inhaled nonsteroidal drugs are available:

- sodium cromoglycate
- nedocromil sodium.

Several oral nonsteroidal anti-inflammatories are currently under development and will be available very shortly. These new drugs belong to a class of drug called anti-leukotrienes, and the first to be launched in the UK is likely to be:

- zafirkulast (Acolate).

Other anti-leukotrienes (and other types of nonsteroidal anti-inflammatory medicine called anti-cytokines) are likely to become available over the next five years or so.

Bronchodilators

The main class of bronchodilating drugs are β-agonists – so called because they stimulate the β-2 receptors in the airway muscles causing the muscles to relax. β-agonists are of two kinds: short-acting (i.e., they last for up to 4 h and long-acting (i.e., lasting for at least 12 h).

Short-acting β-agonists

There are two types of short-acting β-agonist:

- salbutamol
- terbutaline.

The short-acting β-agonists are used for symptom relief, and the efficacy lasts for up to 4 h. They are normally taken in inhaled form, though oral preparations are available.

Long-acting β-agonists

There are two long-acting, inhaled β-agonists:

- salmeterol
- eformoterol.

Long-acting β-agonists are added at Step 3 or above, and these drugs have bronchodilating effects of 12 h or more.

Side effects will be described in Chapter 5; however, it should be noted here that β-agonists will also stimulate, though to a lesser degree, the β-1 receptors in the heart, and so will counteract the effect of beta-blockers and vice-versa.

Other bronchodilators

There is another type of inhaled bronchodilator which works in a completely different manner (it has an anticholinergic effect), of which ipratropium bromide and oxitropium bromide are two examples. These two bronchodilators are more effective in patients suffering from chronic obstructive pulmonary disease (COPD) – some older patients with asthma may also have some degree of COPD.

One final type of bronchodilator, called theophylline, is an oral preparation. This is actually a very old drug, but is now infrequently used and only in low doses as an addition at Step 3 or (more commonly) Step 4 or 5. Because it is an oral preparation, the duration of efficacy can be more than 12 h.

Types of device

Inhaled medicine is provided by means of an inhaler or 'device' which puts the drug into an airborne suspension, and which can be breathed in. There are three mechanisms for achieving this suspension:

1. Metered dose inhalers (MDIs) are aerosol devices containing a solution or suspension of drug particles and a propellant gas.

2. The drug can be prepared in the form of a dry powder which is mixed with air when inhaled. Dry powder inhalers work on this principle.

3. The drug can be added to water which is then 'nebulised' into a fine mist, and the patient breathes in the drug dissolved in the water droplets. Nebulisers work on this principle.

Metered dose inhalers

The metered dose inhaler (MDI) is a bit like a spray can, where the drug is in a pressurised container of drug and gas. The patient presses a button while breathing in through a mouthpiece. Coordination is necessary to ensure that the patient is actually breathing in at the time of button pressing – which is surprisingly difficult for some people.

Whatever the type of MDI, the particles in the gaseous suspension are breathed into the lung, and the small particles tend to get down further than the large particles. Indeed, very large particles simply deposit themselves on the back of the throat, where they do no good. On the other hand the very smallest particles get as far as the alveoli, where they also do no good. It is the medium-small particles which are of greatest benefit.

To overcome the problem of large particles sticking to the throat, a 'spacer' can be used to attract large particles to the side so that only the small particles get into the mouth. A spacer is a bit like a plastic bottle with a hole in the bottom – you breathe in through the top and the MDI is put in at the bottom. The spacer also helps overcome the coordination problem in the standard MDI, because the gaseous suspension remains intact for at least 5 s (the half-life of the drug is about 10 s). The spacer has yet one other advantage. In some patients, the action of an aerosol firing a cold gas into the mouth (with an exit speed of 70 mph) leads to a partial or full closing of the back of the mouth, so that the patient breathes in through the nose. This 'cold freon effect' is prevented by the spacer. Thus, the spacer is a very useful addition to an MDI because it means that the drug gets where it is needed – i.e., in the lung. The disadvantage is that the spacer is cumbersome.

Several new MDIs have been or are currently being launched, including ones which avoid many of the disadvantages of the older MDIs. Developments include breath-actuated MDIs which fire on breathing, thereby avoiding the need for coordination, and MDIs which fire the gas out in a circular vortex, or have a built-in small spacer thereby avoiding the cold freon effect. In addition, the gas in an MDI, which is normally a CFC, is being replaced by non-CFC gases. CFC MDIs will largely be discontinued by the year 2000. The non-CFC gases can be efficient at distributing the drug in the lung. Whereas an old style MDI may lead to a 10% deposition of drug in the lung, the new gases can achieve up to 60% deposition. It is worth noting that CFCs are not harmful to people, only to the ozone layer. However, patients will require education if their device is changed, and in particular because the greater efficiency of drug deposition means that the dose is reduced. A factsheet on CFC-free MDIs may be obtained from the National Asthma Campaign, Providence House, Providence Place, London N1 0NT.

Dry powder inhalers

In the case of the dry powder inhaler, the patient simply breathes in through a mouthpiece, and the action of sucking (which needs to be sufficiently strong) creates the drug–air suspension. The capsule or blister type of inhaler (but not the chamber form) needs reloading once used, and therefore with some models a degree of manual dexterity is needed, though the coordination problem of standard MDIs is avoided, as is the cold freon effect.

As with MDIs, this is an area where rapid advance is taking place. The older devices had the disadvantage that a good deal of the powder became stuck in the throat, leading to an increased risk of side effects. More recent dry powder inhalers were as effective or more effective at getting the drug into the lungs as the standard MDI, and very recent devices are even more efficient, though none as yet is as efficient as the non-CFC MDIs. The consequence is that the effective dose between dry powder inhalers varies, so prescription of dose has to take into account the device used. The new devices are also less cumbersome, and reloading, if needed, is less of a problem.

Nebulisers

A nebuliser is a device containing a plastic reservoir for a solution of the drug plus some mechanism for creating a continuous fine mist of water plus drug – the mechanism is often a compressor but can be an oscillator that creates a high-frequency vibration. The drug for nebulisers comes in the form of nebules – which is a kind of capsule. A nebuliser is a complex and expensive piece of machinery, which is capable of delivering drugs over a longer period of time than inhalers. Although used in acute asthma management, the device is rarely recommended for the management of chronic asthma, though this contrasts with a preference by some patients for this apparatus.

Dose and efficacy

Efficacy of different anti-inflammatories

The efficacy of steroids increases as the dose increases The *British National Formulary* classifies inhaled steroids as either 'standard-dose' or 'high-dose'. Standard-dose inhalers correspond to mild/moderate anti-inflammatories in the commentary on the BTS steps, above, and high-dose to strong anti-inflammatories.

The dose level refers to the amount of drug delivered in any one inhalation. There are several dose alternatives both within the group of standard-dose inhalers as well as the high-dose inhalers. Combining dose level with frequency of inhalation, it is possible to think about dosing as a continuum of mild–moderate–severe anti-inflammatory medicine. The distinction between standard-dose and high-dose or between mild/moderate and strong is therefore simply one of convention, where a continuum is classified by two categories. As a guide, mild/moderate steroids would be anything equal to or less than 500 μg beclomethasone via a metered dose inhaler per day (or equivalent). A typical value for a mild/moderate anti-inflammatory for an adult, i.e., the dose at Step 2, would be a 100 μg beclomethasone MDI with two puffs taken morning and evening (total 400 μg per day), and, for a strong anti-inflammatory, i.e., at Step 3, a 200 μg beclomethasone MDI with two puffs taken morning and evening (total 800 μg per day). However, adult doses can be much higher in the high-dose range, from 1000 to 2000 μg per day beclomethasone by MDI or equivalent. Note that the amount of drug actually deposited in the lung is highly variable because of differences in the technique.

The strongest anti-inflammatory effect is achieved by oral steroids, but these have side effects and so their regular use is reserved only for those patients where asthma can not be controlled in any other way. Oral steroids can, however, be used during exacerbations as a way of achieving rapid control, because their systemic action means that they are assured of reaching all sites in the lung.

The nonsteroidal anti-inflammatories have only mild anti-inflammatory properties, and they should be thought of as 'very mild' rather than 'moderate'. In addition, the ones which have been available for some time (sodium cromoglycate and nedocromil) seem to be effective in only some patients and not others, and their use has decreased considerably in recent years. On the plus side, however, they have a very safe side effect profile. Little comment is possible at this point in time on the new nonsteroidal anti-leukotrienes, but these are likely also to be mild in anti-inflammatory action.

A useful way of comparing steroids with nonsteroidal anti-inflammatory asthma drugs is to use the analogy of a fire. Steroids act like a fire blanket. They put out the fire by swamping everything; everything is put out with one simple action. But the fire blanket can knock things over in the process, and so can cause unwanted side effects. The nonsteroidals, and in particular the anti-leukotrienes (the actions of cromoglycate and nedocromil are poorly understood) act by preventing the fire being lit in the first place. By analogy they act by going round and telling the firelighter 'hey, stop it'. However, fires can be lit in many different ways, and if the particular firelighter is not stopped, then the fire prevention will be inadequate. There are many different types of leukotriene as well as other inflammatory chemicals called cytokines, so, by analogy, there are a lot of firelighters lighting fires, and these nonsteroidals don't necessarily catch them all. It is for this reason that the steroids currently form the backbone of anti-inflammatory asthma medicines.

Step progression and stepping down

The selection of drugs for progression through the BTS steps is shown in Table 1.2 (pp 21–22). The basic principle of management is to increase the dose either within steps or from one step to another until control is achieved. A difference between the earlier and later (i.e., 1997) guidelines is that the latter advocate going in at a reasonably high dose and then reducing (see Ch. 5).

Note that Table 1.2 is designed for adults and schoolchildren, who have half the adult dose. Note also, that the dose levels in Table 1.2 are given for an MDI or equivalent. Other doses may be needed for dry powder inhalers or for MDIs impelled with new propellant gases. However, as a rule of thumb, a commonly given dose for adults at Step 2 is 400 μg beclomethasone or budesonide daily via an MDI; for high dose at Step 3 it is 800 μg beclomethasone or budesonide daily or 400 μg fluticasone daily via an MDI.

The BTS guidelines also allow for patients to be stepped down. The comment given by the BTS guidelines is:

> Review treatment every three to six months. If control is achieved a stepwise reduction in treatment may be possible. In patients whose treatment recently started at Step 4 or 5 or included steroid tablets for gaining control of asthma this reduction may take place after a short interval. In other patients with chronic asthma a three to six month period of stability should be shown before slow stepwise reduction is undertaken.

An additional comment is that stepping down should be considered in the light of any known seasonal asthma – for some patients there are periods of the year when asthma is better or worse.

Pharmaceutical manufacturers and their drugs

When a new asthma drug is discovered, it is granted a patent, and the owner of the patent, i.e., a pharmaceutical company, can then manufacture that drug without competition until the patent expires. When the patent expires, then *any* manufacturer can manufacture and sell that drug, and the drug is described as being *generic*. For example Allen & Hanbury's (now Glaxo-Wellcome) discovered salbutamol which they sold and continue to sell under the name of Ventolin; but the patent has now expired, so that drug is also available from other manufacturers as generic salbutamol. Thus, the same drug may be made available – often with different kinds of inhaler – by different manufacturers, all of whom use different brand names. Consequently it is necessary to distinguish between the chemical name of the drug (e.g., salbutamol) and the brand name (e.g., Ventolin) – which is the name given by the manufacturer to describe their product. As a convention the drug name starts with a lower case letter, whereas the brand name starts with a capital. The *British National Formulary* lists drugs both by drug and brand name, using this convention of capitalisation.

Pharmaceutical companies put a good deal of effort into selling their drugs – i.e., encouraging health professionals to prescribe them. Part of this effort takes the form of demonstrating the advantage of their product over another product, and drug reps will often visit practices accompanied by the latest research evidence supporting their products. However, and as a separate activity, pharmaceutical companies also engage in activities designed to encourage 'loyalty' to their particular brands. For example, they may provide information for patients, in the form of booklets or information guides, though they are not (at least in Europe) allowed to advertise or market their prescribed medicines directly to patients. In addition, companies provide education for health professionals, including practice nurses. Although companies are not allowed, by industry convention, to 'bribe' health professionals by giving gifts, they are allowed to provide educational packages, where the education is provided by an independent expert – and a good meal is also often provided. Drug development and asthma management is a constantly developing science, and meetings of any kind are useful for improving knowledge and skill.

REFERENCES

British Asthma Guidelines Coordinating Committee 1997 British guidelines on asthma management: 1995 review and position statement. Thorax 52(suppl): S1–24

British Thoracic Society, Royal College of Physicians, London, Kings Fund Centre, National Asthma Campaign 1990 Guidelines for the management of asthma in adults 1: Chronic persistent asthma. British Medical Journal 301: 651–653

British Thoracic Society and others 1993 Guidelines for the management of asthma. Thorax 48(suppl): S1–24

Department of Health 1994 Asthma: an epidemiological overview. Department of Health, London

Gregg I, Nunn A J 1989 Peak expiratory flow in symptomless elderly smokers and ex-smokers. British Medical Journal 298: 1071–1072

Griffiths C J, Sturdy P, Naish J et al 1997 Hospital admissions for asthma in East London: associations with characteristics of local general practices, prescribing and population. British Medical Journal 314: 482–486

International Consensus Report on Diagnosis and Treatment of Asthma 1992 National Institutes of Health (Publication No. 92–3091), Bethesda, MD

Kamada A K, Szewfler S J, Martin R J et al 1996 Issues in the use of inhaled glucocorticoids. American Journal of Respiratory Critical Care Medicine 153: 1739–1748

North of England Asthma Guideline Development Group 1996 North of England evidence based guidelines development project: summary version of evidence based guideline for the primary care management of asthma in adults. British Medical Journal 312: 762–766

Effects of asthma on quality of life

2

■ CONTENTS

One of the aims of asthma management is to improve the quality of life of the patient. This chapter describes how patients' quality of life is affected by their asthma.

WHAT IS QUALITY OF LIFE?

'Quality of life' is a phrase used in everyday speech, but it is also used in a more specialised sense in health research. In everyday speech, 'quality of life' is an imprecise term that is used in several different ways, all of which have in common the idea that certain ways of living are 'good'. Good quality of life is associated variously with good housing, high income, safety, happiness or wellbeing, an aesthetically pleasing environment, good health and so on – the list is never ending. People mean slightly different things by 'quality of life', so the use of the term can be ambiguous. Everyone wants a good quality of life, but people do not want the same quality of life. To quote an old phrase: one man's meat is another man's poison.

In health research, the term 'quality of life' is used more precisely and refers to patients' own subjective interpretation of how their health and treatment affects their lives. Patients provide information about their quality of life when they answer the question 'how does having an illness affect your life?'. When patients answer that question they often do so in the terms of the 'gap' between what they would like to do and what they are prevented from doing because of their illness. First suggested by Calman (1984), the concept of a gap between reality and desire has had a major impact on the way health workers interpret the term 'quality of life'. Poor quality of life means that illness has an impact on life as perceived by the patient; good quality of life means that illness does not have an impact on life as perceived by the patient.

One of the implications of interpreting quality of life in terms of 'Calman's gap' is that the perception of the patient is paramount. If, for example, illness has a substantial impact on the patient's life, but *the patient is unaware of this fact*, then the patient, by definition, has a good quality of life. Similarly, if a patient is highly disabled but has very low expectations, then this patient will have a better quality of life, by definition, than a patient with a similar disability but who has higher expectations, and whose expectations are therefore not met. Both these implications may fail to square with commonsense notions of quality of life, and this will be returned to later. Nevertheless, if quality of life is interpreted in terms of a 'gap' between perception and desire (i.e., becomes equivalent to reported dissatisfaction), then quality of life can be represented by a feedback loop showing how people are motivated to close that gap (Fig. 2.1).

According to conventional medical interpretation, quality of life results not only from what is achieved, or, more correctly, *perceived* to be achieved, but also from what is wanted. Whether low levels of wanting *should* imply good quality of life is another matter.

As a general rule, patients try to improve the quality of their lives, i.e., they are motivated to reduce the gap. Sometimes they try to improve quality of life in a way which is not very successful, and sometimes they want a different kind of quality of life to that which the health professional thinks they ought to have. Nevertheless patients do try to obtain the best quality of life, *as defined by the*

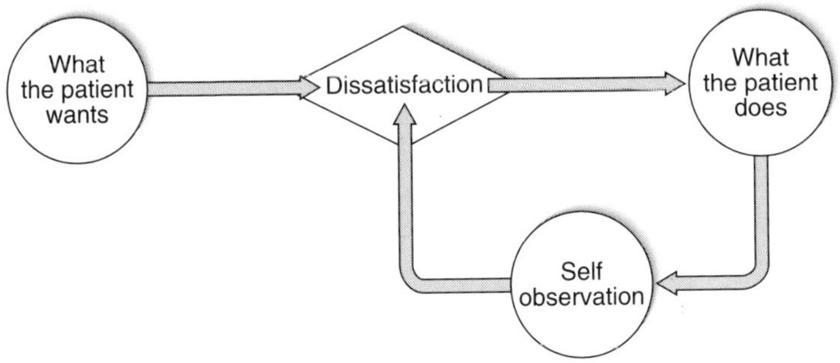

Fig. 2.1 Quality of life represented as a control loop where dissatisfaction results from difference between perception and desire.

patient, achievable within the limitations imposed by circumstances. An understanding of quality of life, or more accurately, different *qualities* of life is therefore a prerequisite for successful asthma management.

A MODEL OF QUALITY OF LIFE IN ASTHMA

A general model of quality of life in disease is shown in Figure 2.2. This model (Hyland 1992a) shows that quality of life is a process involving many different sorts of judgement rather than a single 'thing'. Quality of life is a process resulting from an interaction between two different kinds of variable: physiological variables and psychological variables. The physiological and psychological variables each affect symptoms, problems and evaluations, which are themselves causally connected.

Symptoms

At the left of the model, morbidity (e.g., inflammation and bronchoconstriction) cause symptoms, but whether symptoms are

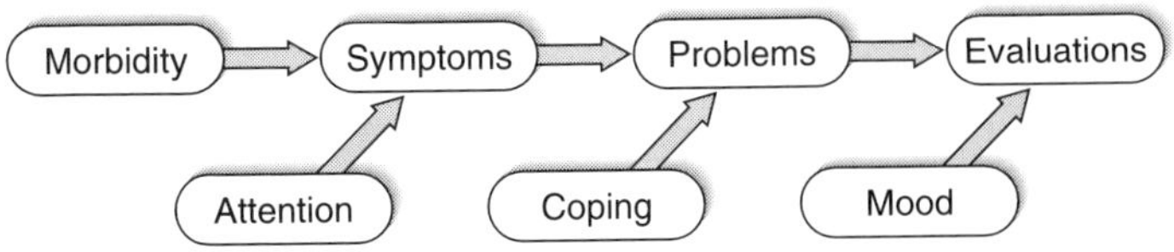

Fig. 2.2 Causal process model of quality of life in disease. From Hyland (1992a).

perceived or not is determined, in part, by psychological factors. Both physiology and psychology contribute to asthma symptom perception, and so asthma symptoms do not correspond exactly to lung function (PEF). Psychological factors can alert the recognition of symptoms in several ways: some patients attend to their symptoms more; others are more anxious about their symptoms and so detect changes more readily (Dales et al 1989); some patients confuse asthma symptoms with feelings of anxiety. By contrast, some patients fail to attend to symptoms or are distracted by outside events or emotions into ignoring their symptoms. Whatever the reason, psychological factors constitute just one of several sets of factors that affect the relationship between PEF and symptoms.

Box 2.1 Attention and symptoms (Pennebaker 1982)

Symptoms are less readily noticed when a person is busy or concentrating on something else. A good demonstration of the way psychological factors affect symptoms is to listen to the amount of audience coughing in a lecture or film. Presumably, the physiological basis for throat tickliness remains the same. However, if the lecture or film is interesting, people cough less. Coughing increases right at the end of the lecture or in the boring bits of a film. Similarly, amateur runners run faster when running along a visually interesting outdoors running track than when they run round a boring indoors running track. The scenery distracts the runners from the discomfort of their symptoms.

Problems

If a patient experiences symptoms, then the symptoms can prevent the patient from doing something, i.e., they cause 'problems', but whether the patient is prevented from doing something depends on the patient's coping style. Some people keep going despite high levels of symptoms. Others stop when they develop symptoms – for example, they go to bed at the first hint of a cold. So the problems experienced by patients depend not only on morbidity and symptoms, but also on other psychological factors having to do with coping style. Health professionals will realise that some of their colleagues soldier on despite being ill, whereas others stay at home and go to bed. In fact, the overall level of absence from work due to illness in an organisation has more to do with staff morale and management than the health of the workers!

Evaluations

Finally, the emotional impact of the illness depends not only on the problems experienced by the patient but also on yet other aspects of the patient's psychology. Some people have a more emotionally positive personality than others; they are 'happy people' irrespective of what happens around them. Some patients with asthma become emotionally upset by their asthma whereas others are much more phlegmatic, and these differences reflect underlying personality differences associated with emotionality.

Illness undoubtedly has an effect on emotional response, but its effect is highly variable because of psychological differences in patients, and these differences can change over time. When accident victims find that they are paraplegic, a common reaction is to be emotionally devastated. During the course of the first year after the accident, this highly negative emotional reaction is often replaced gradually by a more positive reaction where the patient recognises that a good quality of life is possible despite the physical limitations imposed by the accident (Summer et al 1991). In fact, some patients with life-threatening or terminal illnesses report high levels of emotional wellbeing (Evans 1991), often because they have readjusted their goals or approach to life as a result of their illness.

In summary, quality of life refers to a group of judgements people make about their lives. These judgements include the physical

Box 2.2 Well-being

Well-being refers to the general level of happiness of a person. In healthy people, a major proportion of the variance of well-being is the result of personality rather than circumstances (Diener 1984). To put it simply, there tend to be 'happy' and 'unhappy' people. Winning the lottery will not make you happy if you are naturally predisposed to be unhappy (Brickman, Coates & Janoff-Bulman 1978). However, circumstances are not entirely irrelevant, and dramatic changes in circumstances do have effects on wellbeing, though not as much as one might imagine. Hence, trying to win the lottery as a way of improving well-being is not entirely irrational!

problems imposed by illness, as well as the emotional impact of the illness. Physical problems have a causal effect on emotional evaluations, but because of the complex interaction between physiological and psychological variables, physical problems do not always accurately predict emotional evaluations.

HOW PATIENTS DESCRIBE THE EFFECT OF ASTHMA ON QUALITY OF LIFE

Quality of life is a subjective judgement, so the simplest way to find out about it is to ask patients, 'how does asthma affect your life?'. Patients can be asked individually, or they can be asked in 'focus groups' where a group of asthma patients discuss their asthma together. Focus groups have an advantage that the patients stimulate each other to come up with ideas, and the focus group can also be fun for the patient because of the camaraderie and sharing of information. On the other hand, focus groups are not so good at detecting potentially embarrassing problems, such as the effect of asthma on sex.

When describing their asthma, patients' comments fall into three main categories:

1. Asthma causes asthma attacks, and the asthma attack is an unpleasant experience.
2. Asthma causes symptoms, and the symptoms cause problems.
3. Asthma affects quality of life even when no symptoms are present.

Although asthma attacks may appear the most important, these are in fact very infrequent. Asthma mainly affects quality of life when the patient is asymptomatic (normally the majority of the time) or symptomatic. Some patients, including those with moderately severe asthma, never or almost never have an asthma attack. Nevertheless, the effect of an asthma attack, when it occurs, is substantial.

Asthma attacks

Patients report a number of different feelings and sensations when they have an asthma attack. The *Asthma Symptom Checklist* (Brooks et al 1989) is a research tool which was designed to measure experiences during asthma attacks – obviously, the patient does not complete the questionnaire while having an attack, but at some later time. Although the questionnaire is unlikely to be used in normal clinical practice, its items and structure provide useful insight into the experience of an asthma attack.

The Asthma Symptom Checklist has five subscales each made up of several items:

- The Panic–fear subscale includes items describing fear of dying, fear of being left alone, worry about the attack, and feeling scared.
- The Airways obstruction subscale includes items describing the sensation of breathlessness, of congestion and difficulty breathing.
- The Hyperventilation subscale includes items of chest pain, of feeling dizzy and feelings of pins and needles.
- The Fatigue subscale includes items describing fatigue, weakness, exhaustion and numbness.
- The Irritability subscale includes items describing shortness of temper, frustration and edginess.

Not all patients experience all these sensations during an asthma attack, but they are all fairly common to a greater or lesser degree. The important point to note is that asthma attacks are normally accompanied by strong emotional feelings – it is not just a matter of being very breathless – and for many patients with asthma there is a real feeling of fear, a fear which is associated with the feeling of dying from suffocation. Note that a small minority of patients fail to experience strong emotions or severe distress despite having a life-threatening asthma attack.

In addition to the feelings measured by the Asthma Symptom Checklist, patients also comment on how other people react to them when having an asthma attack. A common comment is that onlookers are overly solicitous and 'bothersome', and constantly asking questions like 'are you all right?'. The person with asthma would often prefer to be left alone, and manage the attack with appropriate self-administered treatment. It is not easy to talk when in the middle of an asthma attack, so answering questions is particularly irksome. The person with asthma often knows what to do during an attack and doesn't want other people crowding round, irritating and therefore harming recovery.

If the patient is unable to manage the asthma attack alone, then professional assistance is sought. Reports of emergency care are normally favourable, and the main issue seems to be knowing when to seek assistance or not. Precise description of how to recognise an emergency is therefore important, and is covered in Chapter 4, which deals with self-management plans.

The time between attacks

As already indicated, asthma attacks are rare for most patients, and some will never have experienced one. So for the majority, asthma quality of life is really a matter of what happens at times other than when there is an asthma attack. Most importantly, asthma quality of life is affected even when the patient is asymptomatic. A few examples will illustrate why this is so:

> 'When I go out and visit a friend, I always worry that there may be something there that will cause problems.'
>
> 'Going there the first time is the worst because you don't know what to expect.'
>
> 'You are always aware when other people have colds, and try and keep away from them because you know it affects you.'

These statements illustrate the vigilance asthma patients feel about coming into contact with asthma triggers outside the house. Depending on the particular trigger involved, patients will worry about cats, furniture polish, perfume, or whatever irritates the patient. Broadly speaking, life at home is reasonably controllable, but it is life outside the home which often causes problems.

Life outside the home needs vigilance. If patients have been able to explain about asthma to their friends, life outside the home can become more controllable. Thus, the way others respond to asthma also affects the patient's quality of life.

> 'Well, my friends know about my asthma, so they don't smoke when I am around. They are very good about it. They just say, "Bob's here," and they put their ciggies away.'

Lack of control outside the home is particularly evident when going on holiday. On holiday, there may be a feather pillow or the room may have an air freshener. In addition, asthma patients are away from their normal sources of emergency care, so there is additional anxiety about developing an asthma attack in a strange place. Some patients avoid going on holidays for this very reason of lack of control.

One unexpected place of anxiety is the doctor's waiting room – because waiting rooms tend to be full of people who can pass on their colds. Asthma patients often try and sit as far away as possible from other patients, though this strategy proves useless if someone with a cold comes and sits next to them!

Even with vigilance, some triggers are difficult to avoid, and so the patient's activities are interrupted by the onset of asthma symptoms. In addition, symptoms can arise for no apparent reason. Quality of life can therefore be compromised when the patient is symptomatic even though the symptoms are not sufficiently bad to be classified as an asthma attack. The symptoms have both physical and mental effects. Physical activities are interrupted, slowed down, or have to be abandoned, and the mental effect of the symptoms can be poor concentration, irritability and fatigue.

We have focused on the person with asthma, but society also has a role to play in asthma quality of life. As already stated, the reactions of friends and relations affects quality of life when the person with asthma is symptomatic, but there are also wider social implications. Some asthma patients have a sense of social stigma because they find that having asthma is perceived negatively by others, in particular when it leads to discrimination in employment. Some employers discriminate against people with asthma if the work involves a physical component or isolation (e.g., working on an oil rig). This discrimination can be applied irrespective of the severity of asthma, and the argument that some Olympic athletes have asthma does little to assuage the feeling of unfairness and stigma that this discrimination produces.

A colleague at work once said to me

> 'I have asthma, and I am quite happy to fill in any of your questionnaires if you want – mind you it doesn't affect my work in any way, it really is very mild.'

Why did my colleague find it necessary to deny that asthma affected his work? People only provide an unsolicited denial when they consider the possibility that the opposite may be assumed to be the case. It really wasn't necessary to deny the possible effects of asthma on work in this case – my colleague is much fitter than I am!

In summary, quality of life of asthma patients can be compromised at *any* time – when asymptomatic, when symptomatic and when having an asthma attack. The compromising of quality of life is reflected in two different kinds of judgement made by the patient: physical problems and emotional evaluations. Furthermore, quality of life deficits are also influenced by other people and by values and rules of society.

CLASSIFYING QUALITY-OF-LIFE JUDGEMENTS

As stated above, quality-of-life judgements can be divided into two categories: problems and emotional evaluations. However, these two categories can be further divided, giving a total of four interrelated ways of making judgements about quality of life (Hyland et al 1997), namely:

- activity problems
- avoidance problems
- preoccupation
- distress.

Activity and avoidance are both different kinds of 'problem'; preoccupation and distress are different kinds of 'emotional appraisal'. In the following sections, asthma quality-of-life deficits are reviewed in more depth in terms of each of these different kinds of judgement.

Activity problems

Asthma symptoms can develop because of asthma triggers, or they can develop spontaneously for no apparent reason. Any activity or planned activity may be adversely affected or interrupted when symptoms develop. For example, a patient may become breathless when gardening and have to slow down or stop completely. A patient may be out shopping and have to leave some of the shopping until later. A patient may be at work and find that asthma symptoms cause a loss of concentration or creativity. A patient may go to a party and have to go home early. A patient may play squash and have to stop. Almost any activity can be adversely affected by asthma, including social activities, sport, sexual activity, leisure, home care, paid work and holidays. The particular activities which are adversely affected depend on what the patient likes doing, as well as on the triggers which cause symptoms for that particular patient. For example, ballroom dancing can be a problem for some patients, but not everyone wants to go ballroom dancing; if you don't want to go ballroom dancing, then it won't be a problem! Smoky atmospheres are a problem for many people with asthma: going to a restaurant can be ruined if there are smokers, and some patients find they are unable to visit pubs because of the smoke. Alternatively, it may be the presence of a neighbour's cat which sets off asthma symptoms, or the excitement of a party, or the anxiety of taking an examination. In principle, any activity can be interrupted by asthma symptoms.

Sometimes activities are disrupted by asthma symptoms, and sometimes the activity has to be abandoned altogether. For some activities (for example, housework or shopping) it may be possible to keep going but at a slower rate. In some social contexts, slowing down may be achieved surreptitiously – for example, if, when going out for a walk with friends, one can slow down by 'admiring the view'. Little tricks, like turning round, stopping and saying, 'doesn't the view look wonderful', can be part of a well-developed coping strategy for dealing with breathlessness when in company. Sometimes symptom onset affects concentration, which can be a problem for both manual and nonmanual occupations. Sometimes the onset of symptoms disrupts the enjoyment of an activity, for example, the enjoyment of food or of sexual activity. Sometimes symptoms stop the patient from initiating an activity, making the patient late for appointments or some other preplanned activity.

One way of assessing activity problems is to ask patients to recall what has happened to them during the last week or two. This is a straightforward question to ask, but it helps to ask the question in terms of a definite period of time and to ask for a response in terms of frequency of occurrence. For example:

> 'Did you have to stop doing something in the last seven days because of your asthma?'
>
> 'During the last week how often were you aware of asthma when doing something?'

More specific probe questions can also be used:

> 'Have you been unable to go to work because of your asthma in the last couple of months?'
>
> 'How many times in the last week have you had to stop or slow down when you were walking because of your asthma?'

Some activity problems are embarrassing to talk about, and so patients may not reveal the problem when asked. Sexuality can be an important aspect of quality of life for some people, and asthma symptoms can affect sexual performance as well as sexual enjoyment. The effect of asthma on sexuality may depend on the way the patient's partner responds to the patient's asthma, so sexual response involves more than just the patient. The patient may or may not wish to discuss his or her sexuality, but it is worth being aware that this problem does exist.

Although questions requiring recall of prior events can be very useful, patients can be inaccurate when they try to remember what has happened to them over a period of time, particularly for longer time periods. Memory for the *frequency* of commonly occurring events tends to be poor in all people, both young and old (Raphael, Cloitre & Dohrenwend 1991). The more common and the less emotional the event, the greater is the tendency to forget (Baddeley 1990).

As an alternative to retrospective recall, a structured diary kept by the patient can provide a more accurate record of events. An example of a structured diary is shown in Figure 2.3. Diaries have an advantage in that the effect of memory bias is reduced – though not abolished. If patients are asked to recall the frequency of a problem over a week and their recall is compared with a diary, then some patients underestimate the frequency of the problem. Thus, memory creates a bias so that problems that have occurred are forgotten.

Box 2.3 What is the difference between symptoms and activity problems?

Diary-measured symptoms and activity problems are not equivalent. Activity problems are reported only when there are symptoms, but symptoms can occur without activity problems. A diary study (Hyland & Crocker 1995) where activities, symptoms and PEF were measured showed that PEF on days when there were problems and symptoms was much lower than days when there were symptoms but no problems. Indeed, PEF on days when there were symptoms and no problems was not greatly different from that on days when there were no symptoms. The authors concluded that activity problems represent the troughs in a peak flow graph (Fig. 2.4).

Today's date ....

Please complete in the morning

Please tick ✓	No	Yes
Were you woken by asthma last night?		
Did you have asthma symptoms on waking?		

Please measure Peak Flow ....

Please complete in the evening

Has your asthma caused problems today with any of the following :

Please tick any that apply ✓	Mild	Moderate or severe
Your paid work or study?		
Jobs around the house?		
Social life?		
Personal life?		
Leisure activities?		
Any other problems?		
Any symptoms?		

Please measure Peak Flow ....

Fig. 2.3 Example of a symptom, activity and PEF diary.

One disadvantage of using diaries is that patients can forget to complete them on one or more days – patients are human and humans forget. Because patients often try to please health professionals they can make up entries for missed days. Patients will

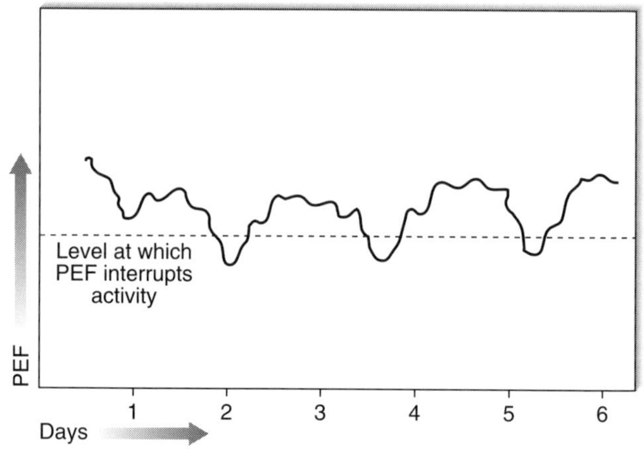

Fig. 2.4 PEF and activity restriction.

sometimes fill in a week's worth of diary entries in the car park before going to the clinic! If diaries are being used as part of clinical assessment, it is best to be open with patients and tell them that forgetting does occur, and that if they forget then they should leave that day blank and just complete the next day. Allowing people to forget makes it less likely that they will lie when they do forget.

Avoidance problems

Humans are good at planning and anticipating events, so it is not surprising that people with asthma anticipate and avoid activity problems. Anticipation of asthma problems is part and parcel of the vigilance many people with asthma have towards their asthma. The experience of asthma relates to the future not just the present. One of the simplest ways of avoiding an activity problem is to avoid that activity completely. A patient can avoid having to stop and rest when going for a walk by not going on the walk. A patient can avoid cigarette smoke-induced symptoms by avoiding places where other people smoke. A patient can avoid the frustration of symptoms developing when doing gardening by not doing gardening. A patient can avoid asthma-related problems at work by registering as disabled and not going to work. Avoidance problems do not arise from specific exacerbations of asthma, but are a way of coping with asthma when the patient is asymptomatic.

In one sense avoidance of asthma triggers is a good thing; indeed trigger avoidance is part of any self-management plan and will be discussed in a later chapter. But the downside is that avoidance may cause the patient to miss experiences because of asthma. Whether 'missing out' is actually a good or bad thing is a value judgement which will depend to some extent on what is being missed. However, patients make their own value judgements. Some patients feel that it is better to have a 'comfortable life' and avoid trouble. Others say they are not going to let asthma get in the way and are going to 'challenge their asthma'. The *balance* between activity problems and avoidance problems is a matter of choice because, for a given level of asthma severity, one can be traded off against the other. Is it better to go to a party and risk an asthma attack or stay at home and watch the television? Is it better to go for a walk or sit at home and knit? Is it better to go into work, even though you are likely to spend most of the morning feeling rotten?

That there is a choice between activity problems and avoidance problems is illustrated in Figure 2.5. Both kinds of problem have emotional consequences, but they have different kinds of emotional consequences. In the case of activity problems, there is the irritation at having to stop something once begun. In the case of avoidance problems, there is the absence of 'life richness' which comes about from being unable to do the same things as others. Often patients make a choice between activity or avoidance problems depending on how the patient interprets the meaning of 'a good quality of life.' This choice is a value judgement and it is possible to make a case either way.

Patients make their own choices about the kind of quality of life they want, but the health professional has a responsibility to help the

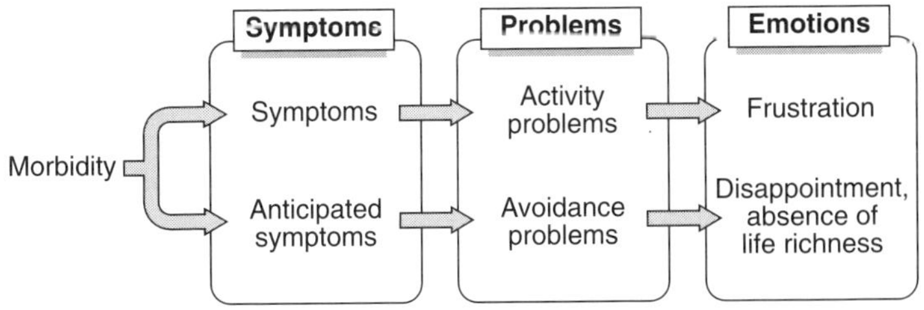

Fig. 2.5 Different types of asthma problem.

Box 2.4 Example of choice between activity problems and avoidance problems

The story of the town and country mouse is a good illustration of the value judgement of choosing a balance between activity problems and avoidance problems. The country mouse invited his city-dwelling cousin to stay with him in the country. However, the town mouse found the food in the country very poor, and suggested that his cousin stay with him in the town where the pickings were much better. In town, the two mice were eating food from a table when they were surprised by a cat and had to make a run for it. The country mouse decided that he preferred the safety of the country even though it meant poorer food.

Neither mouse was 'right'. In the same way, patients make a choice about whether to enter a situation where there is a chance of asthma exacerbation – for example, going to a party – or whether to avoid that situation: for example, stay at home with a good book.

patient make an informed choice. For some patients, avoidance is based on ignorance and fear. For example, a patient may avoid exercise, thinking that exercise is unhealthy because it can lead to asthma symptoms. Such a patient may take more exercise if it is explained that exercise is particularly good for asthma patients, and exercise-induced asthma can often be avoided by taking some bronchodilator immediately before the exercise. Discussion about what patients avoid and why they avoid what they do is a useful precursor to helping patients make an informed choice. Some patients need a health professional's 'permission' to start doing things that they avoid, even though better asthma control means that avoidance is actually unnecessary. Some patients need confirmation that what they want to do or are going to do is all right; by contrast, other patients do it without considering the health professional's opinion. In both cases, discussion and assessment of avoidance problems provides insight into this particular component of asthma quality of life.

Sometimes, patients seem to be completely unaware that they avoid doing things. In one of my first focus groups I asked a group of people with asthma how asthma had affected their lives. One of them said 'Not at all really. In fact, I am not sure why I am here. I don't really have asthma'. However, as the conversation proceeded, it became apparent that this patient had given up work because of asthma, and had moved to the South West of England, because the air there was better for his asthma. Lack of awareness of avoidance is the result of a psychological process called *disengagement* (Carver & Scheier 1990). Disengagement refers to the tendency for a person to 'disengage' from a goal for which there is little chance of success. Disengagement protects people psychologically from the constant reminder of failure, and is neatly summed up by the folk tale of the Fox and the Sour Grapes. When the Fox found he could not reach the grapes, he decided that they were sour anyway. If you can't get something, then you feel more comfortable if you deceive yourself into thinking you never wanted it. In fact, research (Carver & Scheier 1990) shows that an inability to use disengagement is associated with depression, so the Fox in the story had the right approach to life after all!

Although asking people what they avoid can provide useful information for those who have insight into what they are avoiding, for others asking people directly will lead to an underestimation of activities avoided. For such patients it can be more useful to ask them what they do rather than what they avoid doing. Asking patients what they do is quite a good strategy, in any case, as it gives a picture of the lifestyle of the patient. If the patient developed asthma recently, it can also be helpful to find out what the patient used to do before developing asthma, so what they did before can be compared with what they do now.

Avoidance problems can be assessed by asking two different kinds of question which may well produce different kinds of result. The first type of question is:

> 'What sort of things do you have to avoid because of your asthma?'

This question assumes insight into avoidance, which may not always be true, but nevertheless can provide a useful series of responses, e.g.:

> 'I don't go anywhere where it is smoky.'
> 'I try to avoid staying away from home – for example, going on holiday.'
> 'I can't do any gardening.'

However, patients often need to be asked specific questions about what they do or do not avoid, since the general question 'What do you avoid?' is so nonspecific that they need to be cued into specific activities. Another weakness of asking about avoidance is that optimists will tend to underestimate avoidance problems. Some patients tend to 'play down' their problems when talking to health professionals, because it is in their nature not to complain too much.

A second type of question asks patients to describe what they do rather than what they cannot do, for example:

'What sort of things do you like doing in your spare time?'

This kind question is a useful starting point for finding out about avoidance, but it does require further exploration. For example

Question: 'You don't do any sport then'
Patient: 'No, nothing much'
Question: 'Is that because you don't like sport or because of your asthma'
Patient: 'Well both really'
Question: 'If we could sort out your asthma would you start doing sport again?'

In sum, accurate assessment of avoidance is made difficult by the fact that avoidance often reflects a choice patients may have made, and that patients may not have full awareness of the things that they avoid. A combination of different types of questions and general understanding of the patient as a person is the best approach to clinical assessment of avoidance.

Preoccupation

Preoccupation refers to the extent the patient thinks about asthma, in particular with respect to treatment. Many patients report frequent checking that they have an inhaler with them, and some report that finding they have left their inhaler behind can cause asthma symptoms. Some patients say that they are always thinking about their asthma and their treatment, and they are constantly worried about how their health will be in the future. Clearly, over-preoccupation is not a good thing. By analogy, most people care for their teeth by brushing morning and evening, but they don't spend the rest of the day worrying about their teeth. Over-preoccupation leads to asthma having an unnecessary impact on the patient's life, and can also lead to overavoidance. Patients who are high in preoccupation are also high in asthma-specific anxiety, indicated by high levels of fear of asthma attacks. For example, patients who are high on the panic–fear dimension of the *Asthma Symptom Checklist* are likely to be prescribed and use higher levels of medication (Hyland et al 1995) – but they are less likely to need emergency treatment (Brooks et al 1989).

Although over-preoccupation is undesirable, under-preoccupation also has its problems. Some patients are so 'under-preoccupied' with their asthma that they fail to take the medicine correctly. That is, they fail to follow the self-management plan given to them, because asthma is not on the agenda of their lives. Under-preoccupation is particularly associated with denial of asthma, which will be covered in Chapter 6.

It is often the case that health professionals worry only about the under-preoccupied patient, because that patient is at risk for an asthma attack, but over-preoccupation can be damaging for quality of life. The over-preoccupied patient may attend the asthma clinic regularly, learn about asthma in detail, and behave like a model patient, but go home and live a highly restricted life. Preoccupation can be measured relatively easily by asking the patient. The preoccupied patient will readily answer a question such as 'how often do you think about your asthma?'. Answers such as 'All the time' would indicate a particularly high level of preoccupation.

Other statements indicative of high levels of preoccupation include:

'I worry all the time about my asthma.'
'I worry how my health is going to be in the future.'
'I worry about taking all these drugs and how they are affecting me.'

Distress

Distress refers to a general feeling of unhappiness. Some patients report feeling angry with their bodies. They say that they feel that their bodies are out of their control, and they are depressed or made generally anxious about their asthma. Distress refers to a general tendency to be unhappy and to experience negative thoughts when negative circumstances (e.g., asthma) arise. Statements made by people with asthma illustrative of asthma distress include:

'I feel so angry with my body.'
'Having asthma makes me feel so frustrated.'
'I feel I have no control over my body.'
'I feel embarrassed when my chest makes a wheezy sound.'

> 'I don't like the way people look at me when I use an inhaler. I usually go into a toilet if I am somewhere in public.'

Asthma distress is measured by asking patients about their feelings, for example:

> 'What kind of *feelings* do you have about your asthma?'

As a general rule, patients are perfectly happy to talk about their feelings to health professionals, and this tends to be an area which can be neglected in asthma patient assessment if one focuses only on physiological aspects.

DETERMINANTS OF QUALITY OF LIFE

The effect of asthma on quality of life is so variable that there is sometimes little comparison between different asthma patients. Level of physiological morbidity is clearly one factor.

At the very mild extreme of asthma, a patient may have only infrequent symptoms during certain seasons – for example the spring and autumn – or develop asthma symptoms only when having the viral infection of a cold. On those occasions the patient will use a bronchodilator and the symptoms will disappear. Regular treatment for asthma is not needed, and when asthma symptoms arise they are quickly managed with treatment. Asthma is a minor inconvenience that happens from time to time. The patient is unaware of asthma at other times, and the patient may reject the label of 'being asthmatic', and consider the implications of that label for insurance or work purposes inappropriate. These patients interpret their asthma as an acute condition which occurs from time to time.

At the very severe extreme of asthma, a patient takes drugs several times during the day, has put on weight and 'is all puffed out' because of the oral steroids, experiences asthma symptoms and problems almost every day, avoids many situations and activities, misses out on social activity, cannot work, and often has asthma attacks requiring emergency treatment.

In between these two extremes is a range of patients with varying degrees of quality of life impairment, treatment regimen, and risk of asthma attacks. Patients who are at the more severe end, suffer more quality of life deficits, both in terms of activity problems, avoidance problems, preoccupation and distress. Consequently, these different aspects of quality of life are correlated, reflecting an underlying factor of severity. As a general rule, patients who have more activity problems will be more inclined to avoid activities, and will have higher levels of preoccupation and distress.

Although the different components of impairment of quality of life (i.e., activity problems, avoidance problems, preoccupation and distress) correlate with each other, they are by no means perfectly correlated. All four components are affected by physiology and by psychology, but the contribution of physiology and psychology to these different components is not the same. Activity problems tend to be affected more by physiology, whereas distress is affected more by psychology. The reason for this can be seen from Figure 2.2. Problems are more closely connected to morbidity than are evaluations, whereas evaluations (on the right hand side of the figure) are affected by an accumulation of psychological factors which add to the causal sequence. Consequently the correlation between problems (i.e., activity and avoidance problems) and PEF tends to be stronger than the association between evaluations and PEF (Hyland & Crocker 1995). On the other hand, evaluations (i.e., preoccupation and distress) have a stronger relationship with psychological factors than do problems.

Both physiological and psychological factors affect quality of life, but they do so in different ways. Physical problems are affected more by physiology but emotional reactions more by psychology. Health professionals contribute both to the physiology and the psychology of patients, and the asthma clinic is not just a place where only physiological interventions take place. The management of asthma quality of life requires management not only of the patient's physiology, but also of the patient's psychology.

In fact, psychological management of patients has always been important. In the 1920s and 1930s GPs were held in high regard – often more so than today – despite having few drugs to prescribe. There were no antibiotics nor steroids. GPs made up for their lack of drugs by a bedside manner which inspired confidence. In those days GPs dispensed psychological care because they had little physiological care to dispense. The development of more effective physiological treatments has rendered the bedside manner less important, which is unfortunate because quality of life can be altered substantially by good psychological care. Patients can leave the asthma clinic feeling much better about their asthma even though no physiological change has taken place, just as old-style GPs reassure patients just by their presence. A psychological impact is inevitable whenever a health professional interacts with a patient. Communication is not optional. It happens whether or not you speak to a patient. A good 'bedside manner' – or, more commonly, a good 'clinic manner' – helps improve the patient's quality of life even in patients whose drug treatment is optimal

MEASURING ASTHMA-SPECIFIC QUALITY OF LIFE

Purpose of assessment

The easiest way of measuring quality of life is to question patients about their asthma, and to take the time and give the right 'listening' signals. Listening skills are described in Chapter 3, and the kinds of questions that can be used have been described in this chapter. In normal clinical practice, interviews are the most commonly used form of quality-of-life assessment. However, there are occasions when it is desirable to measure quality of life in a more formal way, i.e., by questionnaire. Questionnaires never provide the depth of insight that can be obtained from careful questioning, but they do have their uses, namely:

- They can be used for research purposes as an outcome measure to compare different kinds of treatment. The questionnaire provides a standardised way of questioning patients with quantitative results which can be used in the analysis of a clinical trial.
- They can be used as an audit tool for routine evaluation of quality of care – though most existing questionnaires are too long for this purpose.
- They can be used as a preinterview questionnaire for a later interview. The questionnaire provides preliminary information which can be followed up in greater depth in the subsequent clinical interview.

Quality-of-life questionnaires developed for clinical trials

Three major asthma-specific quality-of-life questionnaires have been developed as outcome tools for clinical research: the Living with

Asthma Questionnaire, the St George's Respiratory Questionnaire, and the Asthma Quality of Life Questionnaire. All were produced in the early 1990s, primarily to evaluate the efficacy of new asthma medicines, and all are rather similar in that patients respond to a series of questions about their lives. The scores from the questions are grouped into domains, or subscales, so that a total quality-of-life score is produced as well as domain subscale scores.

The *Asthma Quality of Life Questionnaire* was developed in Canada by Juniper and colleagues at McMaster University (Juniper et al 1992) and can be used either in an interview or patient-complete format. The questionnaire's 32 items are divided into four domains: activity limitations, symptoms, emotional function, and exposure to environmental stimuli. Copies of the questionnaire can be obtained from Professor E. F. Juniper, Department of Epidemiology and Biostatistics, McMaster University Medical Centre, 1200 Main Street West, Hamilton, Ontario, Canada L8N 3Z5.

The 76-item *St George's Respiratory Questionnaire* was developed in the UK by Jones and colleagues at St George's Hospital Medical School (Jones et al 1992) and has questions divided into three domains: symptoms, activities, and impacts. Copies may be obtained from Professor P. W. Jones, Division of Physiological Medicine, Department of Medicine, St George's Hospital Medical School, Cranmer Terrace, London SW17 0RE.

The *Living with Asthma Questionnaire* is another UK scale developed by Hyland and colleagues at the University of Plymouth (Hyland, Finnis & Irvine 1991) which has 68 questions divided into 11 domains – social/leisure, sport, holidays, sleep, work and other activities, colds, mobility, effects on others, medications usage, sex, and dysphoric states and attitudes – but may also be scored by four domains: activities, avoidance, preoccupation, and distress. Copies may be obtained from Professor M. E. Hyland, Department of Psychology, University of Plymouth, Plymouth PL4 8AA.

Despite having different domain labels, the questions which make up these questionnaires are quite similar. For example, all questionnaires have questions relating to problems and to emotional evaluations. Table 2.1 shows the number of items per questionnaire which ask about problems in each of several areas. However, the questionnaires do differ quite considerably in terms of layout and style of questioning. Each of the scales has been found to be sensitive to change in clinical trials, and each may be used in a variety of

Table 2.1 Estimation of number of activity items for different domains of activity

Domain category	Asthma Quality of Life Questionnaire	St George's Respiratory Questionnaire	Living with Asthma Questionnaire
Social/Leisure	5	5	6
Sport	2	3	3
Holidays	0	0	3
Sleep	2	1	4
Work	9	0	6
Colds	0	1	5
Effects on others	0	4	5
Medication use	0	1	6
Sex	1	1	1
Washing/dressing	0	0	0

From Hyland (1992b)

research contexts where quality-of-life outcome needs to be measured.

Quality of life questionnaire developed for clinical practice

The *Asthma Bother Profile* (Hyland et al 1995) was designed as an aid to clinical practice, and is reproduced at the end of the book (Appendix 1). The questionnaire asks patients to rate 15 bothers associated with asthma, including five activity-related bothers, bothers about the cost and use of medicines, as well as a variety of emotional bothers and concerns. A final section asks patients to rate their asthma care on seven criteria ranging from the need for more information to the perception that the doctor/nurse will respond quickly. Questions about the effect of the cost of medicine and perceptions of the doctor/nurse are important from the perspective of patient management, but not from the perspective of evaluating drug efficacy. Hence these questions are not present in the other questionnaires. The Asthma Bother Profile may be reproduced and used without charge for clinical and noncommercial research purposes.

The Asthma Bother Profile can be used as a preinterview questionnaire which is given to the patient to complete before a clinic visit. It is not necessary to score the patient's responses in any formal way. A simple inspection of responses highlights problem areas and allows the health professional to focus on these areas, if necessary, in the following discussion.

Box 2.5 Comparison of questionnaires

Jacobs & Barnes (1995) showed that the Asthma Bother Profile improves the quality of the interview when used as a preinterview questionnaire. Twenty-seven practice nurses used either the Asthma Bother Profile or the St George's Respiratory Questionnaire as a preinterview questionnaire. 133 patients completed the questionnaire on two occasions in random order. Patients found both questionnaires helpful in describing their experiences, but the Asthma Bother Profile was found to be more helpful. Nurse satisfaction with the consultation and perceived usefulness of the questionnaire was also higher with the Asthma Bother Profile than with the St George's Respiratory Questionnaire.

ACHIEVEMENT VERSUS DISSATISFACTION

Broadly speaking, asthma quality-of-life questionnaires measure *dissatisfaction*. That is, they measure the gap between what patients would like to do and what they are limited to because of their asthma. Whether absence of dissatisfaction is the aim of asthma management is, however, a value judgement. Consider, for example, the case of a patient who is unable to do any gardening because of asthma. Due to the psychological process of disengagement, this patient does not miss gardening, and so does not complain about the effect of asthma on gardening. However, once the patient is put on more effective asthma therapy leading to better control of asthma, then the patient is able to garden, and the patient's wife expects him to do the gardening. However, despite the more effective therapy, the patient sometimes has to slow down when gardening. Hence, the patient starts complaining about gardening, whereas this element of dissatisfaction was missing before the enhanced treatment! Is it better to challenge asthma, even though the challenge will lead to dissatisfaction, or is it better to reduce expectations? Is it better to be a town mouse or a country mouse? Clearly there is no scientific answer – as the answer is a value judgement. However, this example does illustrate a fundamental weakness of asthma quality-of-life questionnaires: they are unable to measure achievement *independently* of dissatisfaction.

A COLLECTIVIST PERSPECTIVE ON QUALITY OF LIFE

Is the individual more important than the group? Societies differ in the value placed on the achievement of the individual versus the achievement of the group (Triandis 1989). In individualistic societies, the individual person's needs are paramount, and society serves only to satisfy those individual needs. In collectivist societies, there is either no distinction between individual and group needs, or if there is, then the individual's needs are considered secondary to those of the group. Western societies tend to be individualistic in orientation, whereas Eastern societies tend to be more collectivist. True collectivism is rare and found only in some hunter-gatherer groups where individual ownership of property is unknown.

The account of quality of life presented above is an individualistic one – reflecting the society in which this book is written. That is, I have considered quality of life only from the perspective of the person with asthma. But what about other people? What about the spouse, children, parents, or friends of the person who has the asthma? Is the effect of asthma on them to be ignored? A collectivist perspective on asthma quality of life can be a useful additional perspective.

The family of people with asthma are affected to a greater or lesser extent by that person's asthma. Family members may become worried by symptoms; their lives may be disrupted in the same way as the person who has the asthma. For example, a spouse may be woken at night, holidays may be restricted, and the spouse may have just as much anxiety about social visits as the patient. Other family members provide an additional perspective on the quality of life of the person with asthma. I have conducted many interviews where the spouse disagrees with the patient's assessment – for example, saying things like 'You are woken much more by your asthma than that, dear. I should know!'. In addition to the effects of asthma on individual family members, having someone with asthma in the family can create an additional economic burden because of the cost of medicines. Effective asthma management can improve not only the quality of life of the patient, but also of family members.

Asthma affects not only families where a family member has asthma but everyone in our society. Days off work are lost due to sickness. Health care resources are limited, and asthma places a burden on those resources. For example, the Department of Health (Department of Health 1994) reports that prescriptions for asthma drugs increased by 80% between 1983 and 1993, and currently account for about 11% of the cost of NHS prescribed drugs – a figure of £350 million in 1993. Undertreated asthma causes unnecessary absence from work leading to lost production. Effective asthma management is needed not only for individuals and their families, but also for society as a whole.

CONCLUDING REMARKS

Quality of life is an important concept in modern asthma care. However, an emphasis on quality of life is not simply a matter of using quality-of-life scales to measure outcome. Nor is it merely an attempt to provide a counterbalance to the rather physiological approach which has characterised some traditional approaches to medicine. Rather, an emphasis on quality of life provides a holistic perspective where the full complexity of subjective judgements made by the patient and the causes of those judgements form the framework for asthma management.

REFERENCES

Baddelely A 1990 Human memory: theory and practice. Erlbaum, London

Brickman P, Coates C, Janoff-Bulman R 1978 Lottery winners and accident victims: is happiness relative? Journal of Personality and Social Psychology 36: 917–927

Brooks C M, Richards J M, Bailey W, Martin B, Windsor R A 1989 Subjective symptomatology of asthma in an outpatient population. Psychosomatic Medicine 51: 102–108

Calman K C 1984 Quality of life in cancer patients – an hypothesis. Journal of Medical Ethics 10: 124–127

Carver C S, Scheier M F 1990 Origins and functions of positive and negative effect: a control-process view. Psychological Review 97: 19–35

Dales R E, Spitzer W O, Schechter M T, Suissa S 1989 The influence of psychological status on respiratory symptom reporting. American Review of Respiratory Disease 139: 1459–1463

Department of Health 1994 Asthma: an epidemiological overview. HMSO, London

Diener E 1984 Subjective well-being. Psychological Bulletin 45: 542–574

Evans R W 1991 Quality of life. The Lancet 338: 363

Hyland M E 1992a A reformulation of quality of life for medical science. Quality of Life Research 1: 267–272

Hyland M E 1992b Quality of life assessment in respiratory disease: an examination of the content and validity of four questionnaires. Pharmaco Economics 2: 43–53
Hyland M E, Bellesis M, Thompson P J, Kenyon C A P 1997 The constructs of asthma quality of life: psychometric, experimental and correlational evidence. Psychology and Health 12: 101–121
Hyland M E, Crocker G R 1995 Validation of an asthma quality of life diary in a clinical trial. Thorax 50: 724–730
Hyland M E, Finnis S, Irvine S H 1991 A scale for assessing quality of life in adult asthma sufferers. Journal of Psychosomatic Research 35: 99–110
Hyland M E, Ley A, Fisher D W, Woodward V 1995 Measurement of psychological distress in asthma and asthma management programmes. British Journal of Clinical Psychology 34: 601–611
Jacobs P W, Barnes G 1995 Asthma clinic questionnaires. British Journal of General Practice, May, 270
Jones P W, Quirk F H, Baveystock C M, Littlejohns P 1992 A self-complete measure of chronic airflow limitation – the St George's Respiratory Questionnaire. American Review of Respiratory Disease 145: 1321–1327
Juniper E F, Guyatt G H, Epstein R S, Ferrie P J, Jaeschke R, Hiller T K 1992 Evaluation of impairment of health related quality of life in asthma: development of a questionnaire for use in clinical trials. Thorax 47: 76–83
Pennebaker J W 1982 The psychology of physical symptoms. Springer-Verlag, New York
Raphael K G, Cloitre M, Dohrenwend B P 1991 Problems of recall and misclassification with checklist methods of measuring stressful life events. Health Psychology 10: 62–74
Summer J D, Rappoff M A, Varghese G, Porter K 1991 Psychosocial factors in chronic spinal cord injury pain. Pain 47: 183–189
Triandis H C 1989 The self and social behavior in different cultural contexts. Psychological Review 96: 506–520

Assessments during initial contact with the patient

3

■ CONTENTS

If patients were all the same, they could all be managed in just one way. As it is, patients are very different, and these differences require assessment, because the provision of a good self-management plan – the topic of the next chapter – depends on assessment. Assessment is needed at all stages of asthma care, but is particularly important when getting to know the patient for the first time, both with people newly diagnosed as having asthma and people with asthma who are being reviewed for the first time.

This chapter covers the basic assessments which should be considered early in contact with the patient and the way that early contact should be set up. More advanced assessments which are needed to individualise self-management plans will be described in Chapter 5.

INITIAL CONTACT WITH THE PATIENT

Forming a therapeutic relationship

Even short contact between two people involves a *relationship*. If the relationship is one of trust and affection, then patients are more likely to be honest and to learn from the health professional. On the other hand, suspicious and authoritarian relationships are unlikely to be therapeutic. There are two reasons why a therapeutic relationship between health professional and patient is important for effective asthma care:

1. Patients are more likely to adhere to advice given by those they like. A good relationship helps compliance, which then leads to effective physiological control of asthma.
2. A positive relationship with the health professional can reduce emotional distress independently of any change in PEF. Patients will feel happier about their asthma, even if there are no physiological changes, just because of their relationship with the health professional.

A few simple pointers will help form a therapeutic relationship early in contact with the patient (Murgatroyd 1985), and, because people make judgements about others very quickly, it is important to establish a therapeutic relationship early on. It is worth reflecting on the fact that interviewers often make decisions about applicants between the second and third minute of an appointment interview (McCormick & Ilgen 1980). Such snap decisions are, of course, very unreliable, but this does not stop people – and patients – making them. The first few minutes with a patient are crucial to the way the patient views you. The effort involved in establishing a therapeutic relationship early on with the patient is always a good long-term investment.

Greeting the patient

1. Smile at the patient. Although this may seem obvious, it is surprising how many health professionals fail to 'look friendly'. For the busy health professional it may be the umpteenth patient of the day. The health professional can feel tired, unwell, or just not feel like smiling. The patient, however, has been waiting for that greeting and it is an important part of their lives. Nonverbal communication sets the tone for verbal communication. A smile is a universal indicator of liking. A warm, friendly smile is an invaluable asset in health care. Of course, it helps if you actually like people!

2. Look the patient in the eye when greeting him or her. Eye contact is a nonverbal signal of liking and interest (Argyle 1975). Avoidance of eye contact (for example, looking at notes while saying 'good morning Mrs Jones') gives the patient a message of lack of interest. Health professionals are particularly prone to avoiding eye contact when they are tired or unwell, so those are times to be particularly vigilant. Eye contact should be maintained when greeting, but too high a level is interpreted as threatening or bizarre. To judge the level of eye contact needed, copy what the patient does: the more the patient stares at you, the more you need to stare back. On the other hand, if they avoid eye contact, possibly because they are shy, then you should not force them to look at you. The level of eye contact should be synchronised with the conversation. Higher levels of eye contact are needed when you end a question, as this signals that it is the other person's turn to start speaking. Reduced eye contact signals that you are about to start speaking.

3. If the patient has not met you before, introduce yourself very briefly and say what you are there for. For example, say 'Hello, my name's Sally Brown; I am the practice nurse and I run the Asthma Clinic here'. This short greeting helps to fill up time when patients are adjusting to you and to the sound of your voice. Patients need a

bit of adjustment time when they 'tune in' to the way you sound, and they also like to know whom they are dealing with. Even if the doctor has already said 'Go and see the asthma nurse'; your saying that you *are* the asthma nurse is by no means a waste. Repetition helps life appear a little more predictable when things may seem unpredictable.

4. Find something which is not asthma related to talk about, i.e., use a bit of small talk. For example say something like 'I see you live in Orchard Close. My mother lives just round the corner. It's nice there isn't it?'. Alternatively, fall back on referring to weather, or say something like 'Did you have to come far?' or 'have you been waiting long?'. It really doesn't matter what it is, but the aim of this nonasthma-related conversation is (a) to show that you are human and the patient can react to you as a human, (b) to show that you are interested in them as a person, and (c) to help reduce anxiety. Some topics of conversation should be avoided, however, and these are: problems with the NHS, problems with the clinic, your own personal problems, and your gripes about the political situation. Small talk on these topics does not engender confidence in the health professional. Listen to the answer given you by the patient – don't appear to rush. The answer will allow *you* to start assessing the patient.

Make sure that the opening comments are positive in one way or another. Possible statements that can be included in the greeting or 'opening gambit' in the conversation include

> 'You have asthma, but it isn't bad asthma.'

or

> 'You have asthma, but we really have such good medicines these days that you won't find it a problem.'

Box 3.1 Order of presentation of information

The order of information presented in an interview affects the patient's perception of the interview. If the interviewer starts with favourable information, then this tends to lead to a more favourable impression than if the interviewer starts with unfavourable information (Peters & Terborg 1975). Hence, it is best to start the interview by saying something positive.

Such reassuring statements are particularly appropriate for newly diagnosed patients, some of whom are traumatised by the diagnosis.

Listening

Research shows that counsellors who say least are often rated as most effective by their clients (Murgatroyd 1985). Forming a therapeutic relationship depends more on listening than on telling. Good active listening skills include reacting appropriately to patient's comments – it is no good sitting still, staring at the patient and thinking nice thoughts. They can't see your thoughts. Maintain eye contact at about the level exhibited by the patient. Nod and make 'um-um' noises. Orient your body towards the patient. Show that what she is saying is having an impact on you. Show sympathy with the sad bits. Laugh at the jokes. Active listening is a skill that requires attention – for the nonverbal cues to work properly you need to pay attention to what the patient is saying. Sometimes patients make jokes as a way of covering up anxiety, and sometimes as a way of expressing a 'hidden question'. A hidden question is where the patient would like to find something out but doesn't know how to ask.

> *Patient*: 'The doctor said it was asthma. Well, got to look on the bright side, it could have been cancer' (laughs).
>
> *Nurse*: 'No' (also laughs). 'Asthma never develops into cancer.'

What the nurse has done is respond in the same way that the patient has presented the conversation (i.e., as a joke), but has cleverly managed to provide information which may possibly be the kind of reassurance the patient wants – but without appearing 'serious and heavy'. Detection and response to hidden questions is a skill that relies on careful attention to what the patient is saying.

Assessing the patient's knowledge of asthma

For the newly diagnosed person with asthma, one of the early tasks is to make sure the patient understands, at least a little bit, about asthma. However, the education needed will depend on prior patient knowledge.

> *Nurse*: 'Do you know much about asthma?'
>
> *Patient A*: 'Well, my son has got it, so I know quite a bit about it.'

or

> *Patient B*: 'It's something to do with nerves isn't it?'

Patients A and B need different kinds of information about asthma. Patient A is likely to be fairly knowledgeable about asthma, and a few additional questions will quickly establish how knowledgeable. An elementary account of asthma for Patient A will appear as though you are talking down, and will irritate. By contrast, patient B has got it wrong, and an elementary account will be appropriate. In addition, patient B's response indicates the need to correct a misinterpretation. Comparison of the information needs of Patients A and B shows that it can be pointless giving information without finding out first what information is needed.

As a general rule, it is useful to establish early exactly how much prior contact the patient has had with asthma and what he or she knows about it. This rule applies not only to the person who has just been diagnosed as having asthma, but also to previously diagnosed patients who are met for the first time. Not every previously diagnosed asthmatic will have had a good asthma education, and some who have had good education will have forgotten it.

Useful questions for the newly diagnosed patient include:

'Does anyone in your family have asthma?'

If the answer is yes, then follow with:

'Do you know what they take for it?'

Other follow up questions include:

'Do they have more than one inhaler?'
'Do you know what the blue inhaler is for?'

Avoid questions that sound like an examination, for example:

'Please tell me exactly what you know about asthma.'

ASTHMA AND SELF-CONCEPT

Reactions to diagnosis

Reactions to the asthma diagnosis can be as varied as the reactions to the news of bereavement – they can involve shock, denial, anger and acceptance – and these reactions can change over time. The way people react to their illness depends on their understanding of what the illness is, what health psychologists call their *disease schema* (Weinman et al

1996). Although health professionals tend to have a schema of asthma equivalent to that described in the first chapter, patients can have a variety of different schema. The patient's disease schema will have a substantial impact on the way the patient reacts to the diagnosis of asthma. Patients who are familiar with asthma – for example, because they have relatives with asthma – are more likely to have a more accurate schema. For those who are unfamiliar with asthma, the schema may simply be a vague feeling of anxiety and unease about the person they have just been told they are about to become.

Box 3.2 Measuring disease schema

The *Illness Perception Questionnaire* (Weinman et al 1996) is designed to measure disease schema, and although it is a research instrument rather than a clinical tool, the structure and questions of the questionnaire provide useful insight into the ways disease schema vary. The questionnaire has five sections:

- *Illness identity* refers to the symptoms that identify the disease. Patients identify a disease in terms of a cluster of symptoms (e.g., wheeze means asthma).
- *Cause* refers to the perceived cause of the disease. Patients often believe that they have identified a cause of their asthma: for example, that it was caused by a virus infection, caused by genetics ('runs in the family'), caused by the environment, or just happened by chance.
- *Time line* refers to the length of time the illness is likely to last. Some patients hope that they will grow out of asthma or that it will spontaneously disappear. Others think that they have it for life.
- *Consequences* refers to how asthma will affect the patient's life. At diagnosis, patients unfamiliar with asthma may have little idea about the consequences, and possibly expect them to be far worse than they actually are.
- *Control/cure* refers to what the patient believes can be done to cure or improve the illness. At the moment, asthma cannot be cured, but this does not prevent the patient's having views that it is curable. The patient's beliefs about control have a crucial effect on compliance with self-management plans.

Some patients say 'asthma really isn't a disease, it's just a condition'. The technical meaning of *disease* and *condition* is irrelevant here. The question is, what do patients mean by these words and why is it important to them to have a 'condition' rather than a 'disease'? The reason for this and similar 'inaccurate statements' stems from a person's need to preserve self-esteem.

Self-concept and diagnosis

Everyone likes to perceive themselves in a positive way, or to have positive self-esteem. It feels good to know that you are a 'good' sort of person (Higgins 1987). The diagnosis of asthma gives information which affects the person in many different ways, one of which is that they see themselves as no longer the 'good' person they were. The diagnosis of asthma is more than just a diagnosis. It tells you about the sort of person you are. It may tell you, for example, that you no longer have a perfect body, or that you are not like your friends. The diagnosis of asthma affects the *self-concept*.

There are several parts of the self. There is the *personal self* and the *social self* (Fenigstein 1987). If asthma is interpreted as a 'chronic, incurable disease' then this affects the personal self – i.e., that the patient has a 'bad sort of body.' On the other hand, if asthma is interpreted as a 'common health complaint' then the threat to the personal self is much less. Some patients need time to adjust to personally threatening information, such as the diagnosis of asthma. Indeed, reaction to the diagnosis of a chronic disease has features in common with bereavement – the patient may need to grieve for the perfect body that he or she used to have.

The diagnosis of asthma can also affect the social self. The patient may consider questions such as, 'How will this affect my job prospects?', 'What will my friends or boyfriend say?', 'What will my mother say?' and so on. The social self is more important to some people (including some adolescents) than others.

For both the personal and social self, it is possible to distinguish the *past self*, the *present self*, and the *future self* (Markus & Nurius 1984). The examples given above refer specifically to the present self, but the diagnosis of asthma can also have implications for the future self. The patient may question, for instance, what implications the diagnosis of asthma has for life expectancy and future quality of life. Younger people in particular evaluate themselves in terms of what they can become in the future, and if asthma affects even unlikely future plans, then the diagnosis has a negative effect on the future or possible self of the patient.

Thus, the diagnosis of asthma has implications for several different parts of the self, but exactly how it affects the self-concept will vary between patients. The diagnosis of asthma affects different patients differently. When patients know that they have asthma, they can preserve their self-esteem, for all their various selves, by minimising the impact of having asthma. The kind of statements involved in this minimisation include:

'I only get asthma sometimes.'
'I haven't really got asthma.'
'I am not actually asthmatic, not really anyway.'
'Anyway asthma is just a condition.'

If, shortly after diagnosis, the patient engages in self-protective denial, it is advisable to avoid 'correcting' the patient. For example, don't say:

> 'On the contrary, Mr Jones, Asthma *is* a disease, a very serious disease, I might add, and over a thousand people die in the UK every year. I would advise you to take a much more serious attitude to asthma in the future.'

I am sure no one would use the corrective statement above, but the intention is to illustrate how such statements can be counterproductive. The therapeutic aim is to keep Mr Jones safe in the short term while he is adjusting to life with asthma, and developing a new disease schema about the nature of asthma. There is no need to assault his self-esteem, as the upset is likely to be much more counterproductive in the long term. People react to assaults on their self-esteem in an irrational way, so such assaults should be avoided. The patient is more likely to respond in the example above with 'silly old cow' rather than 'yes, you are wonderful, nurse, how clever you are'.

In planning care, it is helpful to find out how the diagnosis of asthma affects the patient's self-concept. On diagnosis, some patients need reassurance that asthma is not a major health problem; for others the reassurance is not needed. As changes to self-concept have a substantial affect on mood, monitoring the patient's mood is important at the time of diagnosis and shortly afterwards. If the patient appears to be in shock (little emotional expression, reduced eye contact, behaving on 'automatic pilot') the style of management needed will be very different from that for a patient who is merely concerned to sort out a minor health problem. If a patient appears in shock, then the health professional will need to manage the emotional reaction before starting on practical problem-solving solutions. Patients in shock do not learn well (see Ch. 4). If a highly emotional reaction is suspected, start with a simple question such as 'How do you feel about learning that you have asthma?' Note that there may be a difference between 'having asthma' and 'being asthmatic' for some patients, with the latter sounding worse.

GETTING TO KNOW THE PERSON WHO IS THE PATIENT

In some ways everyone is unique. In some ways, everyone is like everyone else. And in some ways, everyone shares characteristics with some people and not others. Personality is the study of those shared characteristics. Personality does not tell us everything about a person but it does provide a useful framework for understanding some ways in which people differ. There are many dimensions and theories of personality, but those listed below are the most important from the perspective of asthma management.

Neuroticism

What is neuroticism?

One important way in which people differ is in their proneness to negative emotions. This dimension of personality is known technically as 'neuroticism', but the technical meaning doesn't have quite the same connotations as is used in everyday speech. Technically, neuroticism refers to the fact that some people are more prone to autonomic arousal than others when presented with a stressful situation. This tendency to react with emotional lability to stress seems to be a genetic or 'physiologically wired in' characteristic, and causes people to be more prone than others to

Box 3.3 Neurotic

A neurotic person is one who worries a lot, becomes upset by little things, overreacts to situations, tends to see catastrophes lurking round corners, and often feels depressed and anxious.

negative emotions. Emotions such as anxiety, depression and low self-esteem correlate, and are all part of the general trait of neuroticism.

Neuroticism and asthma

Neuroticism is important to asthma in several different ways, one of which is the way it affects quality of life. Quality of life depends not only on physiology but also on psychological factors (see Ch. 2). One of the major psychological determinants of asthma quality of life, particularly emotional evaluation, is neuroticism. People who are high in neuroticism will experience more asthma distress and preoccupation than those low in neuroticism (Hyland et al 1993). In addition, neuroticism affects the patient's behaviour. Some people are 'worriers' – they seem to worry about even trivial matters, including their asthma. Chapter 2 described the high asthma anxiety patient – the patient who is high on the panic--fear dimension of the asthma symptom checklist. Such patients may be overly anxious about their asthma, leading to unnecessary avoidance of activities. Finally, neuroticism may interrupt planned activities, including asthma care, leading to poorer compliance. Depression is related to poorer compliance (Cochrane & Bosley 1994).

Measuring neuroticism

Psychologists assess neuroticism by questionnaire (Eysenck & Eysenck 1991), but questions from these questionnaires can be used verbally, and the patient's answers provide a good guide to whether a person is highly neurotic, highly stable, or (the majority of people) somewhere in the middle.

Questions where the answer will give a perspective on neuroticism include:

'Would you describe yourself as a worrier?'
'Do you sometimes feel rather down about things?'
'Do things upset you easily?'

Positive replies are all consistent with a tendency to neuroticism. My favourite neuroticism question from a questionnaire – though not one which I recommend using in conversation with patients – is:

'Do you sometimes seem unreasonable, even to yourself?'

Patients who are high in neuroticism will show greater emotional lability to asthma, as they will to other stressful life events. People vary in their level of neuroticism: some are very neurotic, some are very stable, but the majority are somewhere in between.

Extraversion

What is extraversion?

Extraversion–introversion is another personality dimension which seems to have a genetic basis, having to do with different resting levels of arousal in the cortex. Extraverts are people who need and seek external sensory stimulation, whereas introverts tend to avoid external sensory stimulation. Extraverts respond badly to situations where there is the potential for boredom. Extraverts tend to be sociable, they like noise and activity. Introverts respond badly to situations where there is too much going on and tend to prefer mental activities rather than those involving external stimulation. Extraverts will become bored sooner when waiting in the waiting room compared with introverts – unless, of course, you provide them with some interesting external stimulation. Introverts do better on jobs which require attention to detail without much change occurring – for example, an aircraft pilot. Extraverts do better in jobs which are always changing and require social contact. Introverts don't like being interrupted when they are working. Extraverts welcome interruptions.

Extraversion and asthma

In arriving at their preferred quality of life, patients can trade off between two different kinds of problem, namely, activity problems and avoidance problems (see Ch. 2). Extraverts will be more inclined to accept activity problems rather than avoidance problems, because avoidance often means that stimulating situations are missed. Good quality of life for the extravert means lots of stimulation, even if, as with the town mouse, that stimulation is dangerous. The extravert is more likely to have activity problems than the introvert. By contrast, introverts are more inclined to accept avoidance problems, because avoidance still allows the kind of mental activity preferred by introverts. Activity problems, however, create stimulation that the introvert is inclined to avoid. Extraverts and introverts respond differently to the quality-of-life problems of asthma.

Measuring extraversion

As with neuroticism, extraversion can be measured by means of questionnaires (Eysenck & Eysenck 1991), and individual questions

Box 3.4 Extravert versus introvert

Here are two patient responses to the question, 'How does asthma affect your social life?':

- *Patient A*: 'Social life! What social life? I have no social life! Since getting asthma, I can't go anywhere where it is smoky. I can't go to the pub. I can't hang around with my mates. It is awful.'
- *Patient B*: 'Well not a lot really. I used to go and play bridge quite a lot, but I find the night air troubles me so I stay at home and read. I really have just as good a time as before.'

from questionnaires can be used in conversation to provide a guide to the patient's level of extraversion. Questions which will give a perspective on extraversion include:

'Do you go out a lot with friends?'
'Are you a very sociable person?'
'Do you prefer to read or study with the radio on?'

(If you ever wondered how some children can possibly do their homework with the radio on, the reason is probably that they are extravert; of course, they may be introvert but just not studying!)

People vary in the degree to which they are extravert or introvert. Some people are extraverts, some people are introverts, and the majority of people are somewhere in between.

Coping style

Coping refers to the way people respond to difficult situations. Whereas the personality dimensions of neuroticism and extraversion reflect general patterns of behaviour, coping can depend to a large degree on context. A person may cope in different situations in different ways. Nevertheless there are broad tendencies for people to cope in a particular manner across a variety of situations, called *coping styles*.

Problem- versus emotion-focused coping

There are two main groups of coping styles: *problem-focused coping* and *emotion-focused coping* (Lazarus & Folkman 1984). A person is said to be problem focused when the intention is to resolve the problem: for example, trying to find a solution to a problem, planning to avoid problems, and finding out how others have solved problems in the past. Note that the problem does not actually have to be resolved: coping refers to the intention, not the success or otherwise of action. A person is emotion focused when the intention is to reduce the emotional discomfort of the problem: for example, complaining to others, distracting oneself with some other activity, denying the problem and getting drunk. Again, coping is defined by the intention rather than by the success of action. A person may try drinking beer to forget his troubles but end up with a headache and feeling depressed, but, nevertheless, the drinking would be classified as emotion-focused coping, because the original intention was to avoid unpleasant emotions.

Coping styles and personality dimensions are not independent. People who are inclined to use emotion-focused coping also tend to be high in neuroticism. In other words, people who are prone to negative emotional experiences are also prone to cope with problems by dealing primarily with the emotional experience, i.e., by emotion-focused coping rather than problem-focused coping.

It is very easy to assume that all patients are problem focused – as many successful people, such as health professionals, are problem focused. Indeed, the design of self-management plans, the holding of asthma clinics and the belief in empowering patients have one thing in common. There is an implicit assumption that the patient is going to deal in a practical, problem-focused way with difficulties arising from asthma once the patient has the correct information. This assumption will be incorrect if the patient's normal mode of coping is to deal with emotional states rather than practical problems Thus, the extent to which a patient is problem or emotion focused will have an important impact on the patient's orientation to the education provided by the health professional.

As stated above, the dimension of problem–emotion-focused coping correlates with the personality dimension of neuroticism. In addition, problem–emotion-focused coping relates to the tendency to approach or avoid difficult situations. Problem-focused copers tend to approach situations and find out more about them. Emotion-focused copers tend to avoid difficult situations and not seek out additional information. In addition, problem- and emotion-focused copers differ in terms of one important motivation: the need for control. Problem-focused copers often try to achieve more control over their lives than emotion-focused copers.

Measuring coping style

Because coping can be situation specific, one should not always assume that coping in one situation is the same as another. However, questions about coping style with regard to asthma can appear a little inquisitorial, and so one may need to ask a slightly oblique question, for example:

> 'If you have a problem, are you the sort of person who worries until the problem is sorted?'

(Answer 'yes' suggests the patient is problem focused; 'no' suggests emotion focused.) However, an alternative approach to assessing coping style is to pay attention to what the patient asks you. Problem-focused copers will respond to a diagnosis of asthma by trying to find out more about it. Emotion-focused copers are more likely to listen to what you say, but not try to find out anything more. Level of interest in finding out about asthma is in itself a useful diagnostic variable. If the patient takes the approach, 'OK, I may have asthma, but let's just forget about it so I can get on with my life', there is a good chance that future coping with asthma will be emotion focused. On the other hand, if the patient is trying to find out the precise details about the side effects of drugs, they are more likely to be problem focused.

Intelligence and memory

Intelligence and memory are both cognitive abilities, and, like other abilities, they vary among people.

Intelligence

There are three types of intelligence: verbal intelligence, arithmetical intelligence and visual–spatial intelligence. An intelligence test (IQ test) provides an average of these different kinds of intelligence, which, although correlated, are not highly related. One person may be high in one type of intelligence but low in another. People who are high in intelligence are able to understand complex ideas more quickly, and hence cope better with complex information.

That said, it is difficult to assess intelligence without formal measurement procedures, and, in view of the variety of different types of intelligence, it is best not to draw conclusions prematurely. Some inference about cognitive ability may be possible from education and occupation, but one should avoid stereotyping people's intelligence on the basis of social class.

Some patients pretend to understand what they have been told, so the question 'Do you understand' does not always provide an honest answer. Patients can pretend to understand for several reasons, including the desire to please the health professional and to avoid looking stupid. Medical knowledge is poorly related to intelligence (Ley 1988). Just because someone appears to be 'an educated sort of person' is no reason to suppose that they know any more about asthma than someone who is less well educated. Knowledge about asthma is more strongly related to prior contact with asthma than to intelligence.

Memory

Memory involves three different cognitive activities: the actual formation of a memory trace, rehearsal of the memory trace to consolidate it into longer-term memory, and the retrieval of that memory trace at a later date. Some people are faster learners than others, and people who are slow learners can have problems at one or all of these stages. Slow learners will need to be told about asthma more gradually than someone who is a fast learner. As with intelligence, it is difficult to assess memory ability without formal tests, and so a practical course of action is to 'test' the patient on asthma knowledge on some occasion after the information was provided. Such tests should be done in a nonpatronising way, and testing should not be made obvious. For example, if a respiratory nurse knows from her notes that the action of bronchodilators and anti-inflammatory inhalers have been explained to the patient, she might ask:

> 'Did I explain how the blue and brown inhalers worked last time you were here?'

This indirect way of asking is much better than appearing to test the patient's knowledge as in an examination. If the patient says 'Yes' to the above question and there is still some doubt about competence, it can always be followed up with:

> 'How much detail did I give you?'

Notice how this second question requires the patient to say something other than 'yes' or 'no'. Such open questions are particularly useful in ascertaining the patient's level of knowledge.

Box 3.5 Dealing with poor memory in a patient

Mrs Smith always seems to understand things she is told in the clinic, but never seems to remember what she has been told from one clinic visit to another. For a period she muddled her brown and blue inhalers and was using the 'reliever' twice per day as she thought the blue one was the preventer. The asthma nurse decided to check up more regularly on Mrs Smith, but also to provide her with a simpler management plan than that normally provided in the clinic.

Everyone has the potential to forget. Older people are often more prone to forget, as there can be a decline in memory with old age. The evidence, however, suggests that this decline is not inevitable and reflects lack of 'mental exercise' rather than a natural biological decline (Baddeley 1996). One should certainly not assume that elderly people are always forgetful, but one should be aware that a certain proportion are.

Social circumstances

Disease severity

Occupational status is one of the best predictors of health status over a wide range of diseases. The lower the occupational status, the more likely a person is to get ill and the lower the average life expectancy. Asthma is atypical in this regard because there is no clear evidence that asthma prevalence is greater in working-class or middle-class families. However, the working-class person with asthma, child or adult, is more likely to have severe asthma (Department of Health 1994).

Consider the following factors which may be relevant. Damp, poorly heated houses are more likely to suffer from mould and the fungal spores associated with mould. Cigarette smoking and hence passive smoking is more common in people from lower socioeconomic backgrounds. People with lower incomes tend to have a less healthy diet.

Compliance

Frequency of emergency treatment is higher in people from less affluent backgrounds, and it is also more frequent in families where there is emotional conflict. Both these factors are thought to be related to compliance, which is covered in Ch. 6.

Assessing social circumstances

Questions about occupational status and education need to be treated with caution, as patients can often find such questions intrusive. Questions about family, on the other hand, are usually accepted as part of casual conversation, and can be introduced at any time when getting to know the patient. 'Do you have any brothers or sisters?' is a much more acceptable opening question than 'What does your husband do?'. The latter question can appear to be evaluative – particularly if the husband is not working or in prison. However, once people start talking about their social circumstances, they often open up and reveal a good deal about their background. In addition, social circumstances can be inferred from locality and type of housing.

PEAK EXPIRATORY FLOW RATE ASSESSMENT

How to take a PEF reading

PEF readings should be taken on diagnosis and for those with asthma who are new to the practice. A reading in the clinic provides the health practitioner with information but also teaches the patient how to use a peak flow meter, or provides a check that the patient knows how to take a reading.

Box 3.6 PEF – instructions to patients

Stand up. Hold Peak Flow Meter horizontally, with scale set to zero. Take a deep breath. Place lips firmly round mouthpiece. Blow out as hard as you can. Repeat three times and take the highest reading.

In taking a PEF measurement, the value obtained by the patient is effort dependent. The procedure assumes that the patient relaxes the inspiratory muscles rapidly. A 'true' reading is based on the fastest exhalation possible by the patient. Hence, if the patient is doing it properly, those three values should be quite similar. The highest reading is taken, because that is the reading which corresponds best to fastest exhalation. If, however, the readings are substantially different, then this raises doubt about the reliability of the method with that particular patient.

PEF can be measured either after or not after the use of a bronchodilator. The bronchodilator will increase the value obtained, perhaps by up to 20%, so it is necessary to check with the patient whether a short-acting β-2-agonist has been taken in the previous 4 h.

Interpreting PEF results

A single clinic-based reading of PEF is useful only if it is added into a calculation. There are two kinds of calculation: percentage-predicted PEF and actual-over-best PEF. Percentage-predicted is a measure of normality of lung function. Actual-over-best is a measure of the degree of asthma control.

Percentage-predicted PEF

To obtain percentage-predicted PEF, the value produced by the patient should be compared with the predicted value for the patient, as given in Figure 1.4 (p. 00).

$$\text{Percentage-predicted PEF} = \frac{\text{Actual PEF} \times 100}{\text{Predicted PEF}}$$

If the patient's actual value is expressed as a percentage of the predicted value, this 'percentage-predicted' value provides a measure of disease severity. Patients with more severe disease have lower percentage-predicted PEF values. For example, a patient with 50% of predicted value has lungs which are only half as good as they should be normally. Hence the percentage-predicted value provides a useful spot measure of how normal the lung function is, on a percentage scale. Asthma medicines restore normality to the lungs, so the percentage-predicted value is affected by both the degree of asthma severity, as well as the control provided by medicines. For example, a value of 85% may arise either because the patient has well-treated but moderately severe asthma or because the patient has mild but poorly controlled asthma.

There are two reasons why the patient's percentage-predicted PEF value should be treated with caution. The first is that PEF is variable over the course of a day (see Ch. 1) and the clinic reading may be different from readings taken at other times of the day. The second is that the 'predicted' value for a patient (i.e., what the patient 'ought' to have) has a degree of imprecision built into it, because of the variety of ways in which people's lung physiology varies. The predicted value is calculated from the average PEF of people of the same gender, age and height as the patient, and there is a degree of PEF variation amongst those people. Nevertheless, percentage-predicted values provides a crude measure of normality – though it is important not to overinterpret the value obtained.

Actual-over-best PEF

Actual-over-best is another way in which a single PEF reading can be evaluated, but it produces a different kind of information about lung function: it provides a measure of control. Actual-over-best is obtained by taking the 'best possible' PEF reading obtained by the patient, obtained preferably within the last year, and expressing the actual value as a percentage of that best value.

$$\text{Actual-over-best} = \frac{\text{Actual PEF} \times 100}{\text{Best PEF}}$$

The value of actual-over-best requires the measure of 'best possible PEF' to be reasonably accurate. 'Best possible' is a theoretical value, because the chances are that the patient is not going to measure PEF when that elusive best measure occurs. Nevertheless, if the patient measures PEF regularly, then the 'best ever' value obtained in a series of readings is sufficiently close to the best possible as makes no difference. Consequently, it is useful to keep a record of PEF in a period of well-controlled asthma – say at least four readings – then the value of best will be reasonably accurate.

Actual-over-best is a measure of control because the value obtained is independent of the severity of asthma – i.e., it is independent of the level of normality (Connolly & Prescott 1990). A patient with actual-over-best of less than 80% is poorly controlled and may need increased medication (the idea of 'action points') based on PEF is addressed in the next chapter). However, patients with severe asthma which is nevertheless well controlled will have values of actual-over-best above 80%.

Diary measures

Because of intrinsic variation of PEF, actual-over-best is affected by the PEF value when the measure is taken, and this fact compromises the accuracy of a spot measure such as actual-over-best. Measurement of PEF on several different occasions, using a diary to record those values, provides a more comprehensive picture of the PEF of a patient. There are three types of measure that can be obtained from diary records of PEF, and which can provide additional information compared with spot measures. Diary measures of PEF should be completed in the morning (on rising) and in the evening (after 6 p.m. but before going to bed), for a period of about a week, and the records can be used to derive the following diary measures:

- average-over-best
- maximum PEF difference
- diurnal variation.

Average-over-best is obtained by taking the average of the morning PEF readings and expressing this average as a percentage of the best. Average-over-best is a statistically more accurate measure of actual-over-best and so is more indicative to the health professional in deciding whether the patient is on the correct step in the BTS guidelines. Values below 80–85% would indicate poor control.

Other calculations

Diurnal variation is the average of the differences between PEF obtained in the evening and next morning. High diurnal variation is an indicator of lack of asthma control or asthma severity – values below 10–15% are found in nonasthmatics, so anything above that value is indicative of some lack of control. Maximum PEF difference is the maximum difference between any two readings during the time of measurement and is also a measure of asthma control.

In addition to these calculations, the experienced health professional will be able to inspect a set or graph of PEF values visually – lack of stability of any kind is a measure of poor control. There is no single gold standard for using PEF to measure either normality or control, and, in fact, the different measures described above are highly correlated. It is common to examine a variety of measures (e.g., actual-over-best, stability in PEF graph, and percentage predicted) and make management decisions on the basis of all the available evidence.

SYMPTOM ASSESSMENT

Symptom assessment involves three components:

1. finding out about the nature of asthma symptoms and the words used to describe them

2. finding out about the severity of symptoms when they occur
3. finding out about the frequency of symptoms.

Symptom words

The asthma symptoms of breathlessness, chest tightness, wheeze and cough were described in Chapter 1, and these are the technical, textbook words that health professionals use. People with asthma, however, use many more words to describe the sensations they have which can be loosely described as asthma symptoms. For example, an investigation (Skevington et al 1997) of the words used by people experiencing breathlessness showed that they could be divided into seven categories of physical sensation (Box 3.7).

Before starting to assess symptoms, the health professional has to check out the *language of symptoms* used by the patient. Communication will proceed more easily if the health professional and patient share the same symptom language, and although many patients quickly learn the medical terminology of the health

Box 3.7 Words used by people experiencing breathlessness

Category	Words
Puffing	A bit puffy
	Puffy
	Puffed out
Asthmatic	Wheezy
	Chesty
Breathless	Out of breath
	Breathless
	Short of breath
Fighting for air	Heavy breathing
	Gasping
	I cannot get air
	Very very difficult to breathe
Pressure	Tight
	Very tight
	Pressing
Choking	Choking
Airless	I cannot get my breath
	Winded
	Ran out of wind

professional, one cannot always rely on patients to change their language to suit that of the health professional! With the newly diagnosed person with asthma, finding out about symptoms is also a way of providing the patient with words which can be used for describing symptoms. When asking questions about symptoms, describe the symptoms in full, so that the patient understands clearly what you mean. For example:

> 'Do you get wheezy – a sort of sound in your chest that you make when you are breathing and you can't stop making?'

As well as questions about breathlessness, the health professional should also ask about night-time waking and early-morning tightness/breathlessness as both are indicators of poor control. Patients should also be asked specifically about cough, because patients can attribute cough to some other cause and so not report it.

Symptom severity

In addition to finding out what words are used by the patient to describe symptoms, the health professional should also try to find out how different words relate to the severity of those symptoms. For example, if the patient uses the words 'breathless' and 'out of breath', then the difference (if any) between the two can be explored by asking:

> 'When you say that you are "out of breath" is this better, worse, or the same as when you say that you are "breathless"?'

The patient can be asked directly about the severity of symptoms: for example,

> 'When your asthma makes you wheezy, is it just a little, or is it very bad?'

Answers to such questions need to be treated with caution because what is bad for one patient is not bad for another. Judgements of symptom severity are affected by a variety of psychological factors, which reduce the usefulness of symptom severity estimates. Optimistic, non-neurotic patients may underreport the severity of symptoms. Anxious, panicky patients may overestimate symptom severity. Indeed, nonasthmatic patients who hyperventilate can present with the same sensations of breathlessness as people with asthma. As a general rule, symptom severity provides less useful information from the perspective of management than symptom frequency.

Symptom frequency

Patients should he asked how often they have the symptoms they describe, but the question should be phrased in terms of a definite time period, and a time period which is not too long. For example, frequency of night-time symptoms may be assessed by a question such as:

> 'How many nights during the last week would you say you were woken by that feeling in your chest?'

Frequency questions should be asked about all the symptoms reported by a patient, and using the symptom language with which the patient is familiar.

Asking the patient to think back over a period of time provides an easy measurement strategy, but there is always the possibility of forgetting and hence underestimation of symptoms, even when a period of only a week is used. Regular, nonsalient events are easily forgotten. If a PEF diary is to be completed, it is worth adding a symptom record on the diary form as well. However, patients who forget about their symptoms are also prone to forget to complete their diaries, so for some patients there is no ideal solution to the problem of forgetfulness. If patients do keep a diary, then invented data are worse than no data, and to prevent the patient completing the diary just before the clinic, it is important to 'legitimise' forgetting. Say something like:

> 'It is very easy to forget to complete your diary every day, and if you do forget, then just leave the day blank and start at the next day. However, do try to complete as much of your diary as possible.'

Standard symptom diaries are available, but the health professional should be aware of the need of individualising these diaries for the symptom language preferred by the patient. Symptom diaries have the advantage that retrospective recall of symptoms may lead to an underestimation of those problems. Note that a symptom diary can be combined with a PEF and quality-of-life diary; an example was shown in Chapter 2.

TRIGGER ASSESSMENT

Questions about triggers

Patients can be questioned about their triggers in two ways: they can be asked about their triggers directly, on the assumption that the patient knows what the triggers are, or they can be asked about situations that cause worsening of symptoms, as a way of helping the patient identify triggers. The first, direct type of question can be tried first, and the second, indirect question used as a possible follow up.

An example of a direct question about triggers is:

> 'Do you know any things that make your asthma worse?'

An indirect question might take the form:

> 'Do you find your symptoms get worse if you go to parties, or in a place which is smoky?'

Sometimes indirect questions may need a careful follow up, for example:

> *Nurse*: 'Does your asthma get worse when cats are around?'
>
> *Patient*: 'Not really, I mean we have two cats and I don't think they make any difference.'
>
> *Nurse*: 'Have you ever had any kittens.'
>
> *Patient*: 'Funny you should mention it, but when one of our cats had kittens, my chest was a lot worse.'

Cats produce dander, but kittens produce much more dander. In the above example, the fact that the patient was sensitive to kittens almost certainly means that cat dander is also an irritant.

Patients' ability to notice triggers or to recognise situations which make their asthma worse depend on there being some variation in contact. However, some triggers are so ubiquitous that patients simply don't recognise that they are having an effect. For example, house dust mite is so common that patients are likely to be exposed to house dust mite faeces most of the time. The same applies to mould spores present in a damp house. Because of the constancy of exposure to house dust mite or mould, the patient fails to recognise the situation causing the asthma symptoms. In addition, the effect of some triggers is long lasting if they increase inflammation, so again, the patient will not notice any difference when in contact or not in contact with the trigger. Finally, some triggers have a delayed effect rather than an immediate effect, making the connection between trigger and bronchoconstriction difficult to identify. For these reasons, one cannot rely on the patient always to identify all possible triggers of asthma. Skin prick tests are available for detecting allergic sensitivity, and a method for detecting occupational asthma using PEF monitoring is described in Chapter 5.

Types of triggers

Triggers can be classified in many different ways. In Chapter 1, they were classified in terms of the underlying causal mechanism. From the point of view of questioning patients, an alternative classification system may be helpful, as follows.

Animals and animal products

Many animals act as triggers for asthma; the most common ones are, in order, cats, dogs and horses, but any pet can have a triggering effect, including birds, gerbils and rats. In a few cases of pet sensitive patients, there is greater sensitivity to one breed of dog than another, and Siamese cats are thought to have allergens distinct from those of other cats. Animal products do not have to be associated with living animals. The feathers in pillows and some soft furnishings, and wool can also have triggering properties.

Household and personal products

Air fresheners, polish, cleaning fluids, and perfumes can all have a triggering effect, with air fresheners and polish being the most common causes of problems.

Plant products

Pollen of various kinds, including tree and grass pollen, flower pollens, weed pollen and, in particular, the pollen of oil seed rape can have a triggering effect. In addition, fungal spores which may, but are not necessarily, associated with woodlands can affect asthma. Some patients have seasonal asthma reflecting the presence of a particular pollen or fungus at that season of the year, so seasonal asthma is often due to plant products.

Indoor air quality

The main household pollutant affecting asthma is house dust mite and, in houses which are damp, mould. House dust mite, the most common allergen in asthma, lives off human scales, lives in soft furnishings, pillows, mattresses etc., and requires a relatively moist and warm environment.

Outside air quality

Fumes from diesel and petrol, as well as gaseous emissions from factories can act as triggers.

Colds and infection

Many patients find that their asthma gets worse when they develop a cold or other respiratory tract infection. Some patients believe they catch colds more easily because of their asthma, and their colds are worse than normal. Some patients notice asthma symptoms just before the onset of a cold.

Industrial products

Many industrial products have a triggering effect on asthma. In addition some chemical products actually cause asthma, the best known being a chemical produced in a particular type of paint spray where a paint and its hardener are mixed just prior to spraying (used in painting cars).

Weather

For some patients it is the ozone which affects them, and ozone at ground level is affected by weather conditions. Ozone in the stratosphere helps keep out ultraviolet light, but at ground level causes respiratory problems. Some patients are more likely to experience asthma-related problems during thunderstorms. Some patients become more breathless when it is windy

Mood

Psychological stress, emotional upset, social conflict, work pressure, and anxiety can all increase asthma symptoms. Asthma attacks occur frequently after a domestic row. Students can bronchoconstrict just before examinations.

Exercise and cold air

Exercise, sometimes in cold air but sometimes just the exercise itself, can act as a trigger. Sometimes patients can exercise in a swimming pool because of the moist air but not on a running track. Sometimes exercise inside a leisure centre is possible but not outside.

Food and drink

Food sensitivity is not thought to be very common in asthma but can be important in some patients. Some foods, such as tartrazine (a yellow dye), nuts, some fish and citrus fruits have a triggering effect which appears 20–30 minutes after eating. Wines and beers can also have a relatively quick triggering effect – though the effect is not due to alcohol which in its pure state is a slight bronchodilator. Other foods, such as eggs, milk and wheat, tend to have a more gradual and delayed effect and may be detected only with difficulty without the use of allergy testing. Sometimes patients who are sensitive to food develop tolerance which disappears when they avoid the food for a while, and reintroduction then causes problems. Asthma exacerbations associated with the reintroduction of a food should be noted as an indicator of a possible trigger.

Sometimes asthma is triggered by the smell of food. Peanuts can have a devastating effect on a small number of patients who are allergic to them – which is a particular problem in aeroplanes as particles from peanuts are readily distributed through the air.

Menstrual cycle

Some women have a pronounced premenstrual dip in their peak flows, normally occurring only in naturally ovulating women (i.e., not taking the contraceptive pill).

Medicines

Aspirin and medicines related to aspirin (nonsteroidal anti-inflammatories) all have a bronchoconstricting effect. Note that oranges and other citrus fruits contain small amounts of this kind of substance. Beta-blockers also exacerbate, both in tablet form and in eye drops

General health status

Although general health status is not itself a trigger, health can influence the extent to which other triggers have an effect. A good diet coupled with regular but not overstrenuous exercise can reduce the effect of other triggers. Being healthy is by no means a bad idea!

RELIEVER MEDICINE USE ASSESSMENT

The frequency of use of reliever medicine (i.e., short-acting β-2-agonists) is one of the most useful assessments in asthma management. Patients commonly use short-acting bronchodilators when they develop symptoms, and so reliever medicine use is an alternative measure of symptom frequency. Note that, very occasionally, patients avoid the use of reliever medicine when symptoms are present (see Ch. 6) but they are very much the minority. Reliever medicine use can be measured in two ways: subjective and objective.

Subjective assessment

Patients should be asked how many times they have used their reliever medicine in a fixed period of time. For example:

> 'How many times a day do you find you need to use your blue inhaler?'
> 'How many times in the last week have you used your blue inhaler?'

However, just as patients may forget symptoms over a period of time it is also possible for them to forget reliever medicine use. In addition, if patients know that they should not be using their reliever medicine more than once per day, they may give the answer which will please the health professional.

Box 3.8 Patient underestimation of use of reliever medication

Inhaler use can be measured objectively by inserting an electronic chip into the base of the inhaler, which records the time and number of presses made by the patient. Using this method, it has been found that almost all patients underestimated their use of reliever medication (Yeung et al 1994). Just asking people to describe frequency of reliever use does not always produce accurate results.

Objective assessment

Reliever medicines use may be assessed objectively by counting the number of prescriptions for the reliever medicine. Reliever medicines tend to be used if they are prescribed, so the method of counting (some surgeries have computerised records, which makes the counting automatic) is reasonably accurate, but it is not sensitive to changes over a short time period. In addition, there is sometimes sharing of drugs between family members who have asthma, so it may be necessary to consider counts for the family as a whole. This point is particularly important if one member of the family has free prescriptions but others need to pay.

ASSESSMENT OF DEVICE TECHNIQUE

The health professional should check the patient's technique by (a) observing inhalation and PEF blowing, (b) asking questions about the order and timing of different inhalers and (c) checking the amount of medicine used against the management plan. Care should be taken not to appear patronising towards the patient. If the health professional starts with the question 'how do you find using your inhaler?' the patient will typically say 'Okay', in which case when the health professional asks for a demonstration the patient may infer that he or she is not being believed. Many patients who are using devices incorrectly think that they are doing so correctly, so it is hardly worth asking them if they are doing it correctly. It is far better to present the checking of technique as a routine procedure, and ask questions afterwards. For example:

'Could you just show me how you use your inhaler?'

(Patient demonstrates)

'Good. ... (straight on to next topic of conversation)...'

Make the 'good' or whatever you say sound routine. Avoid an over drawn 'Well done!' which carries the implication that the patient is an imbecile and you are surprised they got it right.

Devices vary in ease of use but all devices can be used poorly. Underdosing due to poor inhaler technique is surprisingly common.

ASSESSMENT OF ASTHMA BOTHERS

Quality of life and its assessment was described in depth in the previous chapter, and so this section is limited to a few practical points. If the conversation has been focused on disease processes, it may take the patient a moment to realise that the conversation has been switched onto issues which relate more broadly to quality of life. A useful introductory question is

'What about you? Does having asthma bother you much?'

This question can be followed up by looking at the degree of bother and the several different ways that bothers arise. The Asthma Bother Profile (Ch. 2) provides a description of the kind of bothers commonly experienced by people with asthma.

One often neglected asthma bother is the need for more information. Sometimes patients need information because of something they have heard in the media that contradicts what they have been told in the clinic. Media accounts of terrible side effects of steroids can be at variance with what they are told by the health professional – because patients often fail to realise the difference between media accounts of oral steroids and inhaled asthma steroids. Again, finding out *why* patients want information can help health professionals provide the precise kind of information that the patient is seeking.

Box 3.9 Patients' information needs

Research has shown that the majority of patients would like more information about asthma – even when they are attending an asthma clinic (Hyland et al 1995). Often the kind of information they want has nothing to do with asthma management, but rather the way asthma affects people. A patient said 'No one ever told me that going out in windy weather would make me feel breathless'. Of course, not every patient is affected in this way by the wind. One of the difficulties with asthma management is that asthma affects people in different ways. All the many patients who feel that they would like more information actually want different sorts of information, but it tends to be information about 'asthma and life' rather than about the latest advances in our understanding of cytokines.

Sometimes patients start a conversation in the general form of 'Do you think I should do …?', where some activity is specified: for example:

'Do you think I should go and play golf?'

Before replying to this question, it is useful to make a further assessment about what prompts the question – for example, saying:

'What do you think?'

Questions of this nature are seldom unbiased by patient preferences. The patient often would prefer to act in a particular way but needs some help in coming to a decision to act in that way. If one launches in with advice straight away one fails to find out what the patient is actually wanting you to say. Whether you say what the patient wants you to say is, of course, another matter.

One of the consequences of focusing on quality of life is that the assessment becomes more 'patient focused' rather than 'health professional focused'. Although it is necessary to make the assessments that the health professional feels are important, patients also feel that their own concerns need to be properly addressed.

ALLOWING THE PATIENT TO ASK QUESTIONS

The previous section shows that patients may have questions of their own. In addition, patients may have an agenda of their own which is not part of the health professional's agenda. It is important for the health professional to find out what those questions or agenda are. There are two ways of allowing the patient to ask questions: by addressing the issue directly in the clinic, or by providing a written preparation sheet allowing patients to think about questions before coming to the clinic.

Questions in clinic

Questions in clinic of the 'What do you want to know?' variety can sound rather confrontational. A question such as:

> 'Do you have any questions?'

often elicits

> 'No ... no, I don't think so'

as a reply. Questions of this nature can be softened slightly to make them less confrontational, often by a slower, slightly more hesitant delivery but also by the words used For example:

> 'Would you like me to go into a little more detail, on anything in particular?'
>
> 'Is there any thing you hope I might be able to do for you?'

It can also be useful to establish what the patient wants to get out of visiting the clinic. Some patients may see the visit as a chore which you have put in their way for obtaining a repeat prescription. Some are hoping that you will say that they are cured and that they don't need asthma medicine any more. Clearly, the conversation will be more satisfactory from the patient's perspective if you find out what the patient sees as the purpose of the visit. The patient may have travelled some distance, may have waited to see you, and the visit may have interrupted his or her life: it is only reasonable that the patient's agenda is also addressed in the clinic.

Preclinic visit preparation forms

Some patients will not have considered what questions they want to ask before going to the clinic. Indeed, many patients need time to work out what exactly they would like to know. It can be helpful to let patients know that they have the opportunity to ask questions in advance, as this then gives them time to prepare. As an example of giving the patient some warning, one respiratory consultant I know sends patients, with their appointment letter, an information and question form which asks them to write down up to three questions they would like to be answered in the clinic. This approach, which can be adapted in various ways, provides patients with a guide to the kind of services which can be provided by the clinic, and in particular, that information can be asked for rather than simply presented.

Giving patients time to prepare a question to ask the health-professional helps prevent the patient's going out of the door and thinking 'Oh, if only I had remembered to ask X'. In fact, questions asked or information given as the patient is going out the door are often the ones that are most important to the patient. The 'hand on the door phenomenon' refers to the fact that people come out with their real worries when they realise that the opportunity will soon be lost – as they are leaving the room.

Patients are notoriously bad at asking for information, so it is important to make question asking as easy as possible. Sometimes reluctance to ask stems from a concern that the question will make them look stupid; sometimes it is based on the perception that health professionals are busy people and must not have their time wasted; and sometimes it is based on a culture where questions are not asked. Evidence suggests that working-class people find it less easy to ask questions, and they receive poorer care because of it. It is important not to believe in the stereotype that working-class people are less interested in finding out about their disease and treatment.

CONCLUSIONS

This chapter has described several different ways of assessing patients, with an emphasis on assessment made during the first few visits. The assessments range from finding out about the type of person to finding out about lung function, and reflect the belief that an assessment of both physiology and psychology is needed for effective asthma management – as well as an assessment of what the patient actually wants from the asthma management.

REFERENCES

Argyle M 1975 Bodily communication. Methuen, London

Baddeley A 1996 Human memory: theory and practice. Erlbaum, London

Cochrane G M, Bosley C 1994 Compliance with inhaled therapy in asthma. European Respiratory Review 4: 92–94

Connolly C J K, Prescott R J 1990 Pulmonary function and drug regimens in asthmatics. British Journal of Clinical Practice 38: 45–48

Department of Health 1994 Asthma: an epidemiological overview. HMSO, London

Eysenck H, Eysenck S B G 1991 Eysenck personality questionnaire. NFER-Nelson, Windsor

Fenigstein A 1987 On the nature of public and private self-consciousness. Journal of Personality 55: 543–554

Higgins T E 1987 Self-discrepancy: a theory relating self and affect. Psychological Review 94: 319–340

Hyland M E, Kenyon C A P, Taylor M, Morice A H 1993 Steroid prescribing for asthmatics: relationship with Asthma Symptom Checklist and Living with Asthma Questionnaire. British Journal of Clinical Psychology 32: 505–511

Hyland M E, Ley A, Fisher D W, Woodward V 1995 Measurement of psychological distress in asthma and asthma management programmes. British Journal of Clinical Psychology 34: 601–611

Lazarus R S, Folkman S 1984 Stress, appraisal, and coping. Springer, New York

Ley P 1988 Communicating with patients: improving communication, satisfaction and compliance. Croom Helm, London

McCormick E J, Ilgen D R 1980 Industrial psychology. Allen & Unwin, London

Markus H, Nurius P 1984 Possible selves. American Psychologist 41: 954–969

Murgatroyd S 1985 Counselling and helping. Methuen, London

Peters L H, Terborg J R 1975 The effects of temporal placement of unfavourable information and attitude similarity on personnel selection decisions. Organizational Behaviour and Human Performance 13: 279–293

Skevington S M, Pilaar M, Routh D, Macleod R D 1997 On the language of breathlessness. Psychology and Health 12(s): 677–689

Weinman J, Petrie K J, Moss-Morris R, Horne R 1996 The illness perception questionnaire: a new method for assessing the cognitive representation of illness. Psychology and Health 11: 431–445

Yeung M, O'Connor S A, Parry D T, Cochrane G M 1994 Compliance with prescribed drug therapy in asthma. Respiratory Medicine 88: 31–35

Patient self-management plans

4

■ CONTENTS

OVERVIEW OF A SELF-MANAGEMENT PLAN

A patient self-management plan is a set of rules used by the patient to manage his or her asthma. The self-management plan is negotiated between the health professional and patient, after the health professional has provided the patient with information about asthma and its treatment.

There are five activities that need to be addressed when providing the patient with a self-management plan. These are:

1. teaching the patient about asthma as a disease and the action of medicines

2. teaching the patient how and when to take medicines, including the 'action points' for change in treatment
3. teaching the techniques involved in the use of devices – inhalation, PEF measurement and spacers
4. providing the patient with a clear set of guidelines for asthma attacks, that is, when and how to get help
5. teaching the patient about triggers and trigger avoidance.

Two theories in psychology are relevant to all these activities, and these theories will be reviewed before covering the practical details of providing the patient with a self-management plan. The two theories of psychology are:

- theories of empowerment and control – because patients have to manage their own asthma
- theories of teaching and learning – because the health professional has to teach and the patient has to learn.

EMPOWERMENT AND CONTROL

By their very nature, self-management plans empower patients. The emphasis on the *self* means that the patient does some of the managing, and the reason why the patient does the managing is not simply to economise on the health professional's time. Self-management is needed for effective physiological control, as well as having psychological benefits.

Competence motivation

The need for *competence* (White 1959) is an important motivator of human behaviour. Competence motivation – also called effectance motivation or the need for control – refers to the need to feel that you are capable of controlling your environment in ways that are important to you. People are motivated to be competent, effective, or in control of their lives.

Needs are interrelated in the form of a hierarchy (Hyland 1988) where lower-level needs serve to satisfy higher-level needs. The need for competence is one of the higher-order needs, just under the highest-level need, the need for self-esteem. The hierarchical relationship between needs is illustrated in Figure 4.1.

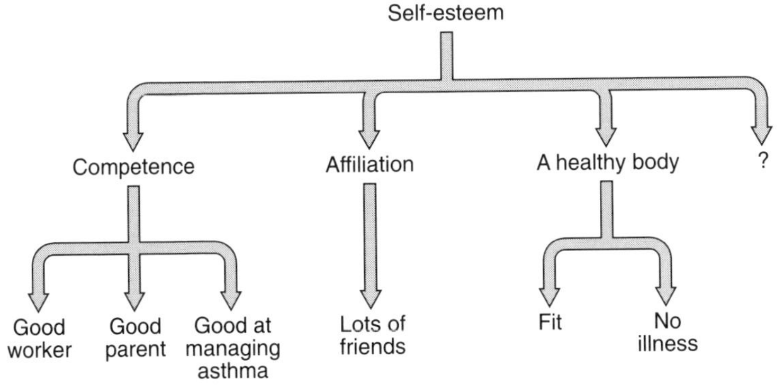

Fig. 4.1 A hierarchy of needs.

Self-esteem can come about in several ways, but most importantly through the satisfaction of needs. For instance, self-esteem comes about by feeling competent, being liked by others, being healthy, and many other needs all of which vary to some extent between people. In fact, we have already discussed the relationship between self-esteem and a healthy body in the previous chapter. The diagnosis of asthma can have a negative effect on self-esteem because it carries the message that you no longer have a healthy body. By contrast, in this chapter, we focus on another cause of self-esteem, the motive for competence.

A sense of competence can be achieved in a number of different ways. For example, one way in which people can get a sense of competence is through their work. Suppose you go home at the end of the day and say to yourself.

> 'I did pretty well today. I sorted out a lot of problems. I sorted them out by myself. I really am good at my job. I am competent. In fact, I really am a wonderful person.'

If you go home saying something like the above to yourself (and I hope you do), then your work gives you a sense of competence, and maintains esteem. In terms of motivation theory (Deci & Ryan 1985), the connection between work, competence and self-esteem means that you are *intrinsically* motivated by your work. Intrinsic motivation leads to greater job satisfaction.

If, on the other hand, you go home at the end of the day, and you say to yourself:

'Well, another £50 in the bank. And I managed to keep out of the boss's way'

then your work does not provide you with a sense of competence or self-esteem. You are *extrinsically* motivated because you are motivated by something (i.e., money) which is outside of the self-concept. Both intrinsic and extrinsic motivation lead to productivity at work, but intrinsic motivation leads to a better *quality* of work produced.

The sense of competence and intrinsic motivation arise not only from enjoying your work. Being a good parent can also lead to a sense of competence, as can any activity which is challenging and which is valued by the person. One other activity which can, but does not always, lead to a sense of competence is the self-management of asthma.

To put it in a nutshell, the aim of asthma management is to get the patient intrinsically motivated so that being good at managing asthma helps the patient's self-esteem. By contrast, the health professional should avoid a management style which encourages patients to be extrinsically motivated, for example managing asthma only as a way of pleasing the respiratory nurse.

All patients have a need for competence or a need to be in control, but some have a stronger need than others. In addition, the strength of the need for control can change over time. When people feel highly traumatised they often want less control than when they are feeling better. A patient may happily relinquish control during an asthma attack but not want to relinquish control at other times. The strength of the patient's need for control is an important factor in developing a management plan, and the strength of this need varies between patients and over time. Quite simply, there is no point in insisting that the patient takes control if the patient won't do so. At the same

Box 4.1 Coping style and control

The differences between problem-and emotion-focused coping styles were described in the previous chapter. People who are high in need for control also tend to be problem focused – because it is often easiest to control things in a problem-focused way. People who are low in need for control also tend to be emotion focused – because they are more concerned with emotions than controlling outside events.

time, there is no point in trying to control a patient's life if the patient doesn't want it.

Variation in the need for control is an important factor when designing a self-management plan. Some patients will want to take control of their asthma; others will want the health professional to be in control. The primary aim of the health professional must always be to ensure that level of control empowerment given to the patient is consistent with the patient's own motivation.

Learned helplessness theory

Learned helplessness theory was first developed in the mid and late 1970s (Seligman 1975) and has had an important impact on the modern approach to patient management. Martin Seligman and his colleagues researched what happens when people find that they are not in control of things that happen to them, i.e., when they are prevented from developing a sense of competence. They found that the lack of control can have wide-ranging psychological effects which were long lasting. The deficits associated with helplessness are:

- motivational deficit – people feel they can't be bothered to do anything
- cognitive deficit – people think less clearly and are less able to work out problems
- sad mood – the feeling of depression
- low self-esteem.

Box 4.2 Learned helplessness research

In one of the early experiments, people listened to unpleasantly loud noise in one of two conditions. In the *controllable* condition, the person could turn the noise off by pressing a button. In the *uncontrollable* condition, the person could not turn the noise off and it just went off by itself. In fact, people in the uncontrollable condition experienced the same duration of noise as those in the controllable condition. After 10 minutes of 'training' with either the controllable or uncontrollable noise, the participants in this experiment were asked to solve anagrams – a problem-solving task which measures cognitive ability. Participants in the uncontrollable condition performed less well on the anagram task than those in the controllable condition. The experience of lack of control had had a long-term effect leading to a 'cognitive deficit' where patients were able to think less clearly.

These deficits were particularly common if people saw the cause of the helplessness to be long term, and saw themselves to blame (Abramson Seligman & Teasdale 1978).

One important finding was that it does not have to be an unpleasant uncontrollable event for helplessness to occur. Positive experiences of helplessness can be just as damaging (Winefield 1983). Whatever the consequences of helplessness, whether it is a positive or aversive event, lack of control can be psychologically unhealthy. Whether or not kindness can actually kill, kindness can certainly lead to poor psychological functioning under some circumstances!

Box 4.3 Positive helplessness

A good example of positive helplessness occurs when someone comes into hospital as an inpatient. Many people have the experience of going into hospital with the intention of reading a lot of books, because going into hospital provides the time which is not normally available in the busy lives we all live. What actually happens? Some reading gets done on the first day. Less reading gets done on the second. On the third day books are abandoned, and all that can be managed are a few articles in magazines. On the fourth day, the person is down to the jokes in magazines. And on the fifth day the person sits staring round the ward like all the rest of the patients!

Learned helplessness can be enhanced by 'kind' carers or health professionals who do everything for the patient, thereby removing any sense of control. Awareness of this problem can help develop strategies to avoid it. For example, learned helplessness can be avoided in long-stay residential units for the elderly by ensuring that residents have choices which affect them – for example, choosing food, what to wear and where to go (Rodin & Langer 1977), rather than having these choices made by 'kind' carers.

However, learned helplessness does not always occur in uncontrollable situations. In the short term, and particularly for people with a high need for control, the experience of uncontrollability leads to *reactance* (Raps et al 1982). Reactance involves increased motivation and activity to try to regain control. In the context of patient care, reactance often takes the form of anger and aggression. The 'difficult patient' is often someone who is experiencing lack of control. Signs of irritation or anger almost invariably have a situational cause: one should not simply assume that anger is because the person has an 'angry personality'.

Learned helplessness is an important concept in asthma management. The erratic development of asthma symptoms can lead the patient to feel helpless, as can a management style where the patient is given no choice. Whatever causes it, a sense of lack of control leads to unhappy patients who manage their asthma poorly. Furthermore, lack of control leads to endocrinological changes (Frankenhouser 1986) and suppression of immune system function (Sieber et al 1992), so it is undesirable for other health-related reasons. Clearly, asthma management should be conducted in a way that minimises feelings of helplessness in patients.

Who is in charge: the patient or health professional?

Health professionals have a need for competence motivation like anyone else. One way in which health professionals can gain a sense of competence motivation is by giving verbal and nonverbal messages that they are 'right'. If the health professional is 'right', then the patient can get the message that he or she is wrong. One potential problem with health education is that the more you tell the patient

Box 4.4 Allowing the patient to be wrong

One piece of advice I give to health visitors is that there are times when they have to allow mothers to be wrong. Mothers almost always feel insecure with their first baby: everyone is telling them what to do. If the health visitor keeps telling them that they are doing things wrong (which is the take-home message when they are told to do things differently), then the mother starts feeling incompetent, and looking after the baby no longer leads to a feeling of self-esteem. As long as the baby is not in danger, it is sometimes better to support the mother in suboptimal behaviour as a way of establishing a good relationship between mother and baby. In the same way, parents have to let go and let their children get it wrong as a way of allowing the children to develop their own sense of competence. Asthma management is no different from parenting. Yes, the patient needs to be educated, but the patient needs to be educated in a way which maintains the patient's competence. The health professional's need to be 'right' must never overshadow the psychological needs of the patient.

that he or she is wrong, the more the patient feels helpless and incompetent. Of course, the health professional may gain a sense of competence by telling others they are wrong, but that is not the aim of health care!

The style of giving instructions can have an impact on the patient's sense of competence. Psychologists distinguish between *informational instructions* and *controlling instructions* (Deci & Ryan 1985). Controlling instructions have the form 'I want you to do ...' and the implication is that the action is being carried out because the communicator is someone in authority:

> 'I want you to measure your Peak Flow when you find you are developing symptoms'

implies that the patient is doing it to please the health professional. Compare that with:

> 'If you measure your Peak Flow when you are developing symptoms, then you will know how your asthma is really doing. That way you can be sure about whether you should change your daily dose of preventer.'

The second sentence provides an informational instruction: instruction is given by way of information, rather than by way of command. Other ways of expressing instructions so they are informational is to use sentences with structures like:

> 'A good way to control your asthma is...'
>
> 'It is so easy to forget, so that what some people find helps is to...'
>
> 'It might be helpful if we reviewed it again in a month's time. It would be interesting to find out how you are getting on.'

Statements which imply control, and so should be avoided with patients who have a high need for control include:

> 'I want to check you are doing things properly.'
>
> 'I want you to follow these instructions carefully.'
>
> Avoid sentences beginning with 'I want you to...'.

In sum, the *self* in self-management emphasises the intention of giving the patient a sense of control in asthma management, and where the level of control given is consistent with the patient's need for control at that point in time. The appropriate level of control should be reflected in (a) the amount of information given to the patient, (b) the nature of the plan itself, and (c) the style of communication.

TEACHING AND LEARNING

All the five activities needed to teach a self-management plan listed at the beginning of this chapter involve teaching. Of course, it is not simply a matter of teaching the patient. The aim is that the patient should learn what is taught (Baddeley 1996). The difference between teaching and learning is crucial. Teaching the patient is a waste of time if the patient is not learning, and the following four general principles of learning can be useful in developing a strategy for teaching what needs to be taught. The four principles are:

1. Learning requires understanding.
2. The more you teach, the more there is to forget.
3. Material at the beginning and end of a list is remembered best.
4. Arousal can harm the learning process.

Principle 1: Learning requires understanding

It goes without saying that patients cannot learn if they do not listen to what you say; and they cannot learn if they do not understand what you say. Patients should be taught in circumstances which are not distracting. Distraction can be external (e.g., other people talking) or internal (e.g., thoughts which the patient produces spontaneously). Sometimes patients want to tell you something which they believe is important for their treatment, and they will not listen until they have got it off their chest. Effective patient assessment (Ch. 2) should ensure that patients do not have a burning message for you which distracts them while you lecture them. External distractions are more obvious to the health professional but may be more difficult to control. External distractions include building noise, radios, other patients, and children.

Accent and dialect can also harm understanding. As a rule of thumb, if you can't make out the patient's accent, he or she probably won't be able to make out yours! *Dialect* refers to the actual words themselves, whereas *accent* refers to the way those words are said. Health professionals have a dialect of their own: it is called medical jargon. Words like 'β-agonist', 'prophylactic', 'bronchoconstriction' are all to varying degrees jargon words which are part of the health professional's 'normal' language, but may be incomprehensible to the patient. Clearly it is important to establish that patients understand the words you use, and one way is to avoid jargon words. As a guide to language use, it is worth reflecting on the fact that writers of leaflets usually design them so that they are understandable by 10-year-old children. Of course, some patients revel in medical jargon and like finding out about correct medical terminology for asthma. The use of simple nonjargon language in these cases can appear patronising, so it is important to be aware of the particular language preference of the patient.

People for whom English is not their native language, or who speak English with difficulty, pose particular problems for asthma education. In some instances family members can act as translators, and if that is the case, particular care needs to be taken to ensure that information is communicated accurately. In some areas of the country, translators are available within the NHS. Cultural differences arising from different belief systems are covered in Chapter 6.

Principle 2: The more you teach, the more there is to forget

It may seem obvious, but there is a limit to what can be learned in a day. There is a considerable amount of information which needs to be taught in the five activities above, and it will not be possible to teach it all in one go. Asthma education should be staged, with the more essential information for the patient's safety being taught first, and other material reserved for later visits. As indicated in Chapter 3, some patients learn faster than others, and so the amount of material given to the patient needs to be tailored to the patient's ability. Selecting the order of material to teach the patient should, as a general rule, be decided by the health professional on a priority basis. Allowing the patient to choose should be reserved for later visits, and particularly for patients with a high need for control.

> 'You will want to know about X and Y, and I can tell you about both, but which would you like me to tell you about first?'

Even if patients learn material in the clinic, they are likely to forget it some time afterwards. In addition, learned material is often recalled best in the context in which it is learned – and the patient needs to remember about asthma at home, not in the clinic. Consequently, it is always good practice to provide (all) patients with a written 'aide mémoire' of what they have been told. This 'aide mémoire' can take the form of a leaflet, or (preferably) a hand-written note where the main points have been written down in front of the patient. A hand-written note provides the patient with a clearer connection between the verbal and written instructions and is preferable for that reason. In addition, the hand-written note can be individualised. However, whether hand-written or not, the patient needs something to take home which summarises the essential features of the self-management plan.

Principle 3: Material at the beginning and end of a list is remembered best

Forgetting occurs for a variety of reasons: one reason is that material which has just been learned interferes with new material which is in the process of being learned; and new material tends to interfere with material which has already been learned. In practical terms, the effect of interference means that the beginning and ends of lists tend to be remembered better than the middle, because the ends suffer less interference.

Try to avoid putting really important information in the middle of a list of material to be learned, as the material in the middle is easily forgotten. If it is logical to put important material in the middle of a list, then repeat it at the end when the patient is about to leave. For example, it may be worth reminding patients that the reliever is coloured blue and the preventer brown as they are leaving the clinic.

Principle 4: Arousal can harm the learning process

Physiological arousal has an effect on memory, and this effect is described by the Yerkes–Dodson law (Fig. 4.2). At very low levels of arousal, the formation of new memory is poor, as it is with very high levels of arousal. The level of arousal which is optimum for learning new information is somewhere in the middle.

Under normal clinical circumstances, memory is more likely to be harmed by overarousal than by underarousal. Patients are particularly anxious when they meet a health professional for the first time, or when they receive a diagnosis, so these times are likely to be less productive for learning than others. In addition, people who are neurotic respond to stressful situations with greater levels of arousal, and so the neurotic person's memory is likely to be particularly damaged by the arousal of a clinic visit.

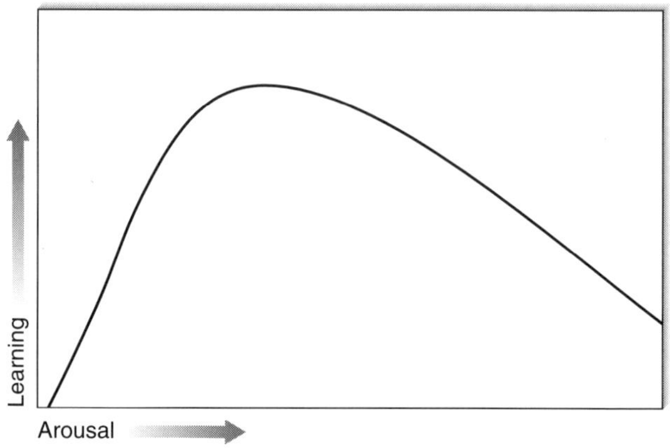

Fig. 4.2 The Yerkes–Dodson law describing the relation between level of arousal and degree of success in learning.

As a rule of thumb, if people appear anxious, traumatised, or in any other way aroused, assume that you may have to repeat what you have just said on a future occasion. Give people time to settle before giving vital information.

TEACHING THE PATIENT ABOUT ASTHMA AS A DISEASE

There are two reasons for teaching the patient about asthma. The first is that information contributes to a sense of control. Knowledge about asthma makes the patient feel less helpless about asthma. The more the patient needs control, the more the patient benefits from information about asthma. The second reason is that information gives a justification for the treatments taken – and consequently increases the likelihood of compliance. Two questions remain: How much and what should patients be taught about asthma? When should they be taught?

All patients need a certain minimal level of education about asthma, but, beyond that minimum, the amount of asthma education needed depends on the patient. As a rule of thumb, patients with higher educational attainment and patients with a greater need for control will need more detail about asthma. The psychological needs and educational characteristics of the patient determine the amount of information to be taught – no routine educational package will be appropriate for all patients.

Because so much information needs to be given, it is not possible to teach it all in one setting – without a high risk of forgetting. Consequently, when staging education over a series of visits, some basic information about asthma should be given on the first visit to ensure patient safety, but other information can be delivered on subsequent occasions.

The most basic information that patients need to be taught is that asthma involves both inflammation and bronchoconstriction, and that treatment is directed at both of these pathological processes. Coloured diagrams and models can be helpful in providing a pictorial representation of these processes

Inflammation

The word 'inflammation' is a technical term but nevertheless is relatively common in everyday language. If there is any doubt about the patient's understanding of this term, an analogy will often help. An analogy is a way of making known something which cannot be seen by referring to something the patient already knows:

> 'Inflammation is rather like what happens when your eyes get red and inflamed. Or have you seen someone with eczema? You know, how the skin gets all itchy and red. Well that's what happens to the inside of the lungs.'

Note that some patients will be made overanxious by too graphic a description of inflammation. Descriptions such as the following should be avoided:

> 'When your lungs get inflamed they get horribly raw and red inside and it really looks a mess.'

Box 4.4 Fear and motivation

Fear does not work well as a motivator. Some of the early anti-smoking advertisements showed pictures of tar-filled lungs in graphic and gruesome detail. These advertisements were found to be ineffective. Communications which induce high levels of fear, particularly in the absence of well-developed coping strategies, lead people to ignore those communications (Janis & Feshback 1953).

It should be explained to patients that there are two types of medicine and that their 'preventer' medicine stops the inflammation. More importantly, they need to understand that the time scale of their 'preventer' medicine is very different from that of the 'reliever' medicine. Again an analogy can help get this message across.

> 'Using your preventer is rather like filling up a large bath which has a small tap and a small plug hole. It takes a while for the bath to fill up, and the bath empties only slowly.
>
> Preventer medicines take a couple of days to take effect (like the bath filling up) and a similar length of time to stop having an effect (like the bath emptying). On the other hand, the action of reliever medicine is like a basin which has a big tap and a big plug hole. The effect of the reliever is very quick – a couple of minutes – but it only lasts up to four hours.'

Patients need to be told the colour of their preventer medicine. It is not that rare for patients to get the 'blue' and the 'brown' inhaler the wrong way round, so this point may need emphasising and checking at a later date. Note that not all manufacturers follow the blue and brown convention, and that long-acting β-agonists can be green or pale blue. The health professional should be aware that the words 'preventer' and 'reliever' are not actually very informative to a person with newly diagnosed asthma. Perhaps the 'preventer' prevents symptoms getting worse and so should be taken when needed, and the 'reliever' relieves inflammation and so should be taken regularly.

Depending on the patient's level of awareness and concern, and after the basic notion of inflammation has been grasped, it may be necessary to bring up the issue of the side effects of steroids. It is important to emphasise that what the patient should be told depends crucially on what the patient has heard and believes about steroids, so initial assessment (see Ch. 3) is essential. If, because of familiarity with asthma, the patient does not believe inhaled steroids to be

Box 4.5 Distinguishing preventer and reliever

It can be useful to write down for the newly diagnosed:

- Brown = preventer = twice daily, regularly = prevents inflammation
- Blue = reliever = when needed = relieves tightness.

harmful, then there is no reason to raise the issue of side effects. However, for patients unfamiliar with asthma, there is a good chance that they will have heard the word 'steroids' used in some negative way – even if it is just something about athletes taking steroids. For these patients and for patients who are 'steroid phobic', a *balanced* argument needs to be presented. A one-sided argument (e.g., 'steroids are perfectly safe') in this context will be less believable.

Self-evidently, steroids have dangerous side effects. There is no point in trying to deny this fact. If one denies that steroids are dangerous then the health professional's advice will appear inconsistent with information already received – and so unreliable. The health professional should explain to the patient that the dangerous side effects are associated with oral steroids, and even these are not dangerous for short periods (up to three courses of 7–10 days per year), as limited use does not have any lasting impact. The point to get across is that excessive doses of steroids are dangerous but the level of dose and mode of administration of inhaled steroids is very different from those for oral steroids, and it is for this reason that inhaled steroids are safe for people with asthma. Dry powder blisters and capsules are useful for demonstrating the small amount of drug used.

Once the issue of side effects has been raised, patients will want to know what those side effects are, and if this information is not given, imagination will attribute every symptom, related or unrelated to asthma, to steroids. It should be explained that side effects are extremely rare but depend on dose (see Ch. 5 for details). The most common side effects noticed by the patient are oral Candida, sore throat and hoarseness, and, with high doses, skin thinning leading to easy bruising. (A puffed out face only occurs with regular oral steroids). These side effects are readily observable by the patient, so if the patient knows what they are, and knows that they do not occur in his or her particular case, then this may go some way to reassuring the patient about the safety of steroids. In addition, patients should be told that none of these side effects is dangerous. They are more of an inconvenience. Patients worry about danger more than inconvenience. Sometimes health professionals are reluctant to inform or ask about side effects, because they believe such information will stimulate greater recognition of those effects. Although asking direct questions about side effects certainly increases the rate of report, it is unclear why this happens. It may be that prior to asking, patients failed to recognise and report symptoms; or it may be that asking about symptoms induces patients to imagine symptoms which are not actually there. It may be one for some patients and the other for others. However, the interpersonal advantage of being open with the patient about side effects far outweighs any over-reporting that may occur in a small minority of cases. Anything less than complete honesty will be interpreted as the health professional's trying to hide something – and they will assume that you are hiding something far worse than you are.

Additional information about inflammation can be added, either for more advanced 'students' who want more information about their asthma, or simply because the patient asks. The additional information includes:

- the fact that inflammation is a self-perpetuating cycle because the byproducts of inflammation cause further inflammation; consequently, the body cannot 'heal itself'
- that there are nonsteroidal anti-inflammatory medicines, and the effectiveness of these should also be discussed
- that the inflammation results from overactivity of the white blood cells, and many different types of white blood cell are involved
- that inflammation leads to production of mucus, epithelial shedding and mucus plugs
- that inhaled steroids mimic the body's own steroids which are a response to long-term stress, but also occur in low doses in all people every day – more being produced in the morning than the evening.

Bronchoconstriction

The terms 'bronchoconstriction' and 'bronchodilation' are technical terms and should be used only with patients who are knowledgeable or have a preference for technical language. The patient should be taught that there are muscles in the airways, which 'squeeze the tubes making them narrower'.

The words 'muscle spasm in the lungs' conveys the meaning of bronchoconstriction, and 'medicines which relieve muscle spasm' conveys the meaning of short-acting β-2-agonists. Patients should be taught that asthmatic airways are more twitchy than normal airways, that twitchiness can be made worse by inflammation, that triggers cause muscle spasm bronchoconstriction and that 'relievers' relieve the muscle spasm.

> 'Asthmatic airways are more "twitchy" than normal. They tighten up when you breathe in small particles like you get in smoke.'
>
> 'They tighten up when you breathe in dirty air, but the reliever medicine makes the airways relax so the air flows through normally.'

Patients should be told the colour of their reliever, to take their reliever when needed, and that a couple of puffs should to the trick. They should be told that if they are having an asthma attack then they should take a number of puffs – specified for the patient – and taking lots of puffs will not damage them in any way (25–50 puffs of salbutamol, 15–20 puffs of terbutaline).

Patients should be taught that reliever medicines have few side effects, other than tremor, pounding heart, headaches, facial flushing, and that overdosing is not dangerous. Patients should also be told that frequent use of relievers (i.e., if needed at least once per day) shows that there is uncontrolled inflammation, so if they are using a lot of reliever, they should come back and discuss this with the health professional.

Patients with a high need for information can also be told that reliever medicines are similar to adrenaline, which is a short-acting stress hormone naturally produced by the body, and that the effect lasts for no more than about 4 h.

Other information

Patients should be taught about any other drugs they are using (e.g., anticholinergics, theophyllines, long-acting β-agonists), but only if they are using these drugs, again using a language which is suitable for the individual patient.

If the patient is the sort of person for whom increased information leads to an increased sense of control, then a variety of additional information about asthma can be given, even if it has no relevance to the patient's treatment. Such information could include the epidemiology of asthma, cross-cultural differences in asthma prevalence, and the puzzle of what is causing the increase in asthma incidence and prevalence. None of this information will help management – but it will provide a greater sense of control for those patients who want it. If the patient is very curious about asthma, he or she should be referred to a good textbook on the subject – popular texts are readily available from booksellers and libraries. Asthma patients with a positive attitude towards education in general will often want to be educated about asthma. It is worth noting that popular books about asthma are often read irrespective of advice from a health professional, and a large number of them include material on complementary medicines for asthma.

TEACHING THE USE OF DEVICES AND *HOW* TO TAKE MEDICINES

There are two kinds of knowledge: factual knowledge and procedural knowledge. Factual knowledge is knowing about things – for example, knowing who is the prime minister. Procedural knowledge is knowing how to do things – for example, knowing how to ride a bicycle. Teaching about asthma as a disease and the action of asthma medicines (i.e., the previous section) requires the patient to learn factual knowledge. But learning how to use devices requires procedural knowledge. Procedural learning needs a different kind of approach compared with informational learning. In the case of informational learning, the student can learn it from a book, or from verbal instruction. In the case of procedural learning, it is far better to *see* what has to be learned, and then to copy it. Procedural learning is most effective when the learner can 'model' himself or herself on the teacher. In practical terms, this means that when teaching patients about devices, the best way is to show them. Although written instructions of 'how to do it' can be helpful, they are no substitute for seeing how it is done. You cannot learn to ride a bicycle from a book. The health professional should keep a selection of placebo medicines, as well as spacers and PEF meters to demonstrate to the patient, and after demonstrating how it is done, ask the patient to practise. The health professional should demonstrate techniques with an accompanying verbal description. For example:

> 'You breathe in and hold your breath for 10 seconds, like this.'
> 'This is how you put in a new disk/capsule.'

Once the patient has learned the procedure for device use, there is additional factual information which can be added. The following advice can be given as appropriate.

- Don't polish the spacer with a cloth. Polishing creates a static charge which attracts particles. It is better to just rinse it out and leave it to drain.
- Some inhalers malfunction when stored in a damp environment such as a bathroom.
- Each device provides some kind of information about when to get a new prescription – some better than others – and patients should be showed what this is.

One feature of procedural knowledge is that, once well learned, it does not get forgotten. People don't forget how to ride bicycles even if they have not been on one for several years. However, device design is changing much faster than bicycle design, and new devices imply new procedural learning. In addition, you will not be able to ride a bicycle after one session, so one should not assume that one session of training with an asthma inhaler leads to effective use of the device. Thus, one needs to check that patients are able to use their device correctly, but once they are doing so then checking is probably unnecessary.

Inhalation technique is often poor. The points to pay particular attention to for MDIs are: (a) shaking inhaler before use; (b) coordination of actuation and breathing, i.e., beginning to breathe in just before actuation; (c) not closing the back of the mouth and breathing in by the nose (cold freon effect); (d) breathing in steadily rather than very fast. The point to pay particular attention to for dry powder inhalers is: breathing in sufficiently fast to create a good

Box 4.5 Is the MDI still working?

MDIs often give poor feedback about when they are about to run out. MDIs can be floated in water – they float when nearly empty. Some patients say they are able to work out how full the MDI is by its feel and sound when shaken. However, many 250-dose MDIs continue to function after the 250 doses have been administered, but the doses given after that point tend to vary in amount. Patients may think that they are having adequate inhaled steroids when they are not.

dispersion of drug. The points to pay particular attention to for all devices are: (a) breathing out fully before inhalation, (b) breathing in fully, and (c) holding the breath for 5–10 s (authorities vary on this figure) after inhalation.

TEACHING THE PATIENT WHEN TO TAKE MEDICINES

Level of control

Let us start by assuming that the patient has been prescribed a particular regimen according to the BTS step system, and that the patient needs to take regular prophylactic medication. In addition, the patient needs to *self*-manage, i.e., control the timing and modification of dose. However, not all self-management plans give the same amount of control to the patient. In practice, a good deal of the variation between self-management plans reflects the health professional's view of 'patient empowerment', but ideally such variation should be tailored to the individual needs of the patient. Consider the following three approaches to a Step 2 patient:

1. The patient should be on a sufficiently high dose of inhaled steroid to avoid any exacerbations. If the patient 'needs' to increase the steroid dose from time, then the patient is on an insufficiently high regular dose of steroid.
2. The patient should be on an adequate regular dose of inhaled steroid for most occurrences, but on certain occasions (e.g., when developing a cold or when particularly exposed to a trigger) than the patient should increase the dose.
3. The patient should be on the minimum dose of inhaled steroid for most occurrences, but on certain occasions (e.g., when developing a cold or when particularly exposed to a trigger) then the patient should increase the dose. In addition, when the patient is in a good phase, then the dose can be decreased.

In case (1) there is no variation in inhaled steroids under patient control. In case (2) there is moderate variation in inhaled steroids. In case (3) there is substantial variation in inhaled steroids. The degree of control given to the patient increases from (1) to (3).

From a psychological perspective neither (1), (2) nor (3) is 'right' for all patients and at all times. However, each strategy may be 'right' for particular patients at particular times. For example, (1) would be appropriate for patients with poor memory, poor coping skills and a low desire for control; (2) would be appropriate for people with an average desire for control; and (3) would be appropriate for knowledgeable people with a high desire for control and who want to manage their asthma with a minimum level of steroids. Although I have no hard evidence to support this, my experience is that health professionals who have asthma (including consultants and respiratory nurses) tend to opt for (3) in their own cases, even if they advise patients otherwise.

Box 4.6 Do as I say, not as I do

When I give talks to health professionals on the psychology of asthma management, I often start the talk by asking people in the audience to put their hands up if they have asthma. Up to a third usually do so. I then ask them how many manage their asthma by taking regular and consistent prophylactic medicine. Hardly anyone ever raises their hand!

There is no rule for how much control should be given in a self-management plan, since each patient should be treated as an individual. Patients who feel traumatised by their asthma – including people newly diagnosed with asthma – may be more comfortable with a plan that gives relatively little control. However, the degree of control given to the patient may need to be reviewed, since with increasing confidence the patient may prefer a pattern of self-management that provides greater empowerment. Patients with

Box 4.7 Desire for control in a self-management plan

A survey carried out by the author (Hyland 1997) illustrates that patients can either want more control or less control in their self-management plan than they are actually given. Patients were asked whether they had been told to increase the 'brown inhaler' by the doctor/nurse when symptomatic, and whether they would do so. They were also asked whether they had been told to reduce the dosage when their symptoms were better and would they do so. As will be seen in Table 4.1, most patients said they did what the doctor/nurse told them to do. But some patients had a more complex and some a simpler pattern of managing their asthma.

Table 4.1 Number of patients responding to questions about increasing or decreasing their brown inhaler when more or less symptomatic

		Patient would increase		
Doctor has said		**No**	**Not sure**	**Yes**
increase	No	14	5	6[a]
	Not sure	1	2	2
	Yes	4[b]	0	80
		Patient would reduce		
Doctor has said		**No**	**Not sure**	**Yes**
reduce	No	36	5	12[a]
	Not sure	2	1	4
	Yes	17[b]	6	30

[a] These patients are taking more control than they have been given.
[b] These patients are taking less control than they have been given.

problem-focused coping styles, who are knowledgeable and confident in their asthma management, are likely to respond better to a self-management plan which provides greater control – and will exert that control if it is not offered. Thus, the level of control provided in *self*-management needs to be adjusted to different patients, and for any patient over time.

Giving instructions for action points

In terms of specific instructions, patients should be told how many puffs of their preventative inhaler, and how many times a day. The instruction to take it 'when you get up in the morning and when you go to bed at night' is quite helpful, but one may need to check whether the patient is a shift worker.

Box 4.8 Case study

One patient who took part in one of my studies consistently failed to take her evening preventer. The patient was a farmer's wife who had a variety of other health problems. When I asked her why she wasn't taking her medicine, this is what she said. 'The nurse says I have to take the second lot after six o'clock, and as I sometimes go to bed before six o'clock, I can't take the second lot.' The nurse had given the right advice, but not the right advice for that particular patient.

Instructions to increase the dose of inhaled steroids or to start a course of oral steroids should be given verbally as well as written down. The patient should be given *precise* information about when to increase dosage – for example, when PEF drops to a certain level, or when the patient feels a cold is coming on. The patient should know exactly what to do as a function of symptoms or PEF, and the instructions should be adjusted to the circumstances of the patient.

You will note from the example in Box 4.9 that there are two 'action points' in this plan. The first action point is at a PEF value of 400, when the patient is told to increase dosage; the second action point is at 250, when the patient is told to contact the doctor. A commonly used way of representing action points to the patient is through the use of the 'traffic light' zone system. For example, according to international guidelines (International Consensus Report 1992), when PEF is above 80% of best the patient is in the 'green zone' and should continue with treatment as normal. When the patient is between 50% and 80% of best, then the patient is in the 'yellow zone' and should increase steroid treatment. When the PEF is below 50% of best, the patient is in the 'red zone' and should seek assistance. The precise figures for these action points (i.e., 80% and 50%) are somewhat arbitrary. For instance an action point of 70% for

Box 4.9 Example of instructions on dosage

Here is an example of instructions that may be given to a male patient with a best PEF of 500. The example is illustrative only, since all advice, including PEF values, depends on the individual patient (see Ch. 5).

> 'You should normally take two puffs in the morning and two in the evening. If your PEF ever falls below 400, then double your dose of preventive medicine: that means, four puffs in the morning and four puffs in the evening. Keep going at the doubled dose until your PEF gets above 400 again.'
>
> 'If your PEF drops below 250, then you must contact the doctor the same day, and preferably straight away. Contact the doctor immediately on 123123, and if you can't get through, telephone 321321 instead.'
>
> Note how in this instruction the meaning of 'doubling the dose' is made explicit, and the health professional has anticipated that the normal telephone surgery number may sometimes be constantly engaged.

steroid increase is recommended by one group (Beasley, Cushley & Holgate 1989). The positioning of action points will be discussed in the next chapter.

Preparation for forgetting

If a patient is on regular prophylactic therapy (as above), it is almost inevitable that the patient will forget to take his or her medicine on one or more occasions. It is human to forget. The self-management plan should therefore have an instruction for what to do when forgetting occurs. The issue of forgetting needs to be made explicit – otherwise the patient will make a guess and the guess may be wrong.

As steroids have a gradual onset and offset of effect on inflammation, the effect of missing one dose of steroid is not very drastic. Inhaled steroids are, comparatively speaking, a 'forgiving drug' because the patient is not greatly at risk from a short period of forgetting. By contrast, anti-hypertensives are not forgiving, because a relatively short period of forgetting leads to an increase in blood pressure, putting the patient at risk. However, steroids are not so forgiving that the patient can forget on one day or more without the likelihood of an increase in inflammation. Hence, patients should be advised that if they forget their prophylactic medicine on two or more occasions, then an additional dose of inhaled steroid should be taken next time. Of course, this will be sensible advice in some but not all cases. If the patient's level of medication is comfortably adequate to control the inflammation, then a longer period of time can elapse without any increase in inflammation. The extent to which steroids are 'forgiving' of forgetting will depend on the individual patient.

Although missing an inhaled steroid on an odd day may not have any great physiological consequences, there can be psychological consequences if the health professional takes too 'laid back' an approach to forgetting. If the health professional gives the message 'It doesn't matter too much if you forget' then this can lead to the interpretation 'It doesn't matter too much if you stop'. An example of advice which creates a more appropriate balance is:

> 'If you find you forgot to take your medicine on one occasion, don't worry as long as it is just the one occasion. Just take your medicine at the next evening or morning. However, if you forget (two, three or whatever is appropriate for the patient) times, then take an extra couple of puffs next time, because your inflammation will be starting to creep up.'

Note how, in this example, the issue of inflammation is introduced at the end of the sentence, where it is likely to be remembered best.

Although some forgetting is inevitable, patients should be advised about ways to avoid forgetting – for example, by placing the inhaler somewhere where it will be seen when getting up and going to bed.

PROVIDING THE PATIENT WITH GUIDELINES FOR ASTHMA ATTACKS

All patients have the potential for an asthma attack. Asthma attacks are difficult to predict and may take the form of a gradual decrease in PEF – which allows time for remedial action – or a rapid decrease. Knowing when and how to call for assistance in an emergency is a crucial part of asthma management. It is essential to avoid the possibility of ambiguity, and, as far as possible, patients should be given very precise instructions. What may be clear to the health professional, may not be clear to the patient so careful attention to communication is needed. For example, do not say, 'if you have an asthma attack, you had better contact us', because the patient may not actually know what an asthma attack is. Other words which are potentially ambiguous are 'emergency' and 'urgent'. For some patients it is only an emergency when they are about to fall unconscious. For others it is an emergency when they start feeling rather worried. Advice should be given using words where there is little scope for multiple interpretations.

Patients should be advised to take their bronchodilator if they experience worrying symptoms (20–50 puffs salbutamol, 15–20 puffs terbutaline), and to adopt a relaxing and calming position (relaxation should be practised in advance; see Ch. 5). The patient should try to use tidal diaphragmatic breathing, with relaxed muscles (shoulders down), which reduces oxygen needs. (Note that deep breaths require more energy than tidal breathing.) Sitting slightly forward on a chair is a good position, but lying flat on the back is not good, as the internal organs add weight to the diaphragm. Loosening tight clothing may help.

The patient should be advised to seek help if the normal bronchodilator fails to have an effect a short time after use when acute symptoms are present. However, the 'short time after use' needs to be specified exactly, as does the use of the bronchodilator, and the degree of benefit. Commonly, the patient is advised to wait 5 min before seeking assistance, though in fact most short-acting β-agonists should have an effect after 2 min. The following is an example of an instruction:

> 'If you are breathless and find that you are getting worse, then take about ten puffs of your reliever. If after four minutes you do not find that you are *definitely* getting better, then you need emergency help.'

Note that the health professionals should not say 'you are getting a little better' or just 'getting better' – as this carries the risk that the patient imagines improvement when none is present. The patient needs to recognise a definite improvement, rather than imagine a small improvement.

The BTS guidelines suggest that patients need emergency care when PEF drops below 50% of best. This is a useful guideline for patients as it provides an objective criterion for seeking assistance, particularly in the case of gradual decreases in PEF. However, patients may not have a PEF meter handy when an attack develops, and it is important that patients are not put off calling for assistance because a PEF meter is not available.

Box 4.10 Severe or life-threatening asthma attacks. Features of *severe asthma* requiring treatment by a health professional include:

- PEF equal to or less than 50% of best
- too wheezy or breathless to complete a sentence in one breath
- respiratory rate of 25 breaths per minute or above
- a heart rate of 110 beats per minute or above.

Features of *life-threatening asthma* requiring immediate transfer to hospital include:

- PEF less than 33% of best
- exhaustion, confusion, or coma
- feeble respiratory effort
- lips turning a blue colour
- bradycardia or hypotension.

Note: patients may not be overly distressed either with severe or with life-threatening asthma. Any of the features above should alert the health professional to severe or to life-threatening asthma.

The patient should then be given a number of actions in the event of an asthma attack, which will depend on the circumstances and location and capacity of the patient. The following points should be considered:

- How far is the patient's home from a hospital accident and emergency department? To what extent does the clinic need to provide an emergency service?
- Has the patient a car or normally has access to a car? If not, how should the patient respond, and in any case how should the patient respond if the normally available car is not working?
- If the patient is telephoning the clinic, what number should be used and what should the patient do if that number is engaged or is not answered? There can be a difference between how a practice manager understands telephone contact to work, and how the patient experiences it. Patients may need to be told, for example, 'If after three minutes you can't get through on the number I have given you, then dial 999'.
- Does the patient have a relative or partner who should also be involved in setting up emergency courses of action, and if so how are they going to be informed about what to do? Does the patient have a telephone in the house or flat?

Emergency response by the patient should be written down in an easily accessible format – when the patient is having an asthma attack, he or she is likely to be cognitively impaired and therefore need all the help available when decision making. Some patients have a natural tendency 'not to make a fuss', and such patients may think 'let's leave it just a little longer; I might get better'. A clear, precise instruction will prevent such patients putting their lives at risk.

In setting up a sequence of actions for emergency care, plans need to be made for the variety of different places away from home that an attack may occur – travelling, at sea, etc. To explore this, it is useful to ask the patient

> 'Is there anything I may have missed? Is there any situation which has not been covered?'

In addition to providing a plan for seeking assistance, the health professional should consider any medication advice to give to the patient. Inhaled steroids are not recommended during an asthma attack, because an inhaled steroid penetrates more slowly into the lungs when lung function is very poor (though I have heard informal reports that if nothing else is available they can be helpful). Some patients are provided with oral steroids for emergency use, and taking oral steroids when an attack seems imminent may help. However, it is important that seeking assistance is not delayed when it is needed.

In summary, the essential feature of the emergency action plan is that *every* eventuality is covered, and covered very precisely so there is no ambiguity as to how the patient should react. The 'if–then' rules for emergency action need to be individualised. Although it would be more convenient if patients had similar lives, the reality is that they don't and what may work with one patient does not always work with another. When you tell a patient 'telephone if …' consider the possibility that the patient may be too embarrassed to admit not having a telephone. Ask before telling patients how to react in an emergency.

TEACHING THE PATIENT ABOUT TRIGGER AVOIDANCE AND TRIGGER MANAGEMENT

What acts as an asthma trigger for one patient may not affect another, so assessment of triggers (Ch. 3) is the first step in providing advice about trigger avoidance. There are two psychological considerations in teaching patients to avoid triggers.

1. The recognition and avoidance of triggers introduces an element of control into the patient's experience of asthma. That is, it reduces the sense of learned helplessness which may develop if the patient interprets the asthma as something which happens to him or her in an unpredictable way. Trigger recognition and avoidance is, from this perspective, psychologically healthy, and should be encouraged.
2. Trigger recognition and avoidance can encourage an avoidant coping style which has negative effects on quality of life – and so trigger recognition and avoidance should be discouraged.

In practice, the health professional – and the patient – need to balance these two considerations. It is possible to avoid some triggers without any appreciable loss in quality of life, but most trigger avoidance will involve the patient in some kind of choice. The following examples illustrate the choices involved.

- *House dust mite*. House dust mite can be reduced by avoiding wall-to-wall carpeting, and using rugs on floor boards, or cork tiles, or linoleum or other forms of non-absorbent flooring – but some people like wall-to-wall carpeting. House dust mite can be reduced by keeping all windows open when vacuuming – but this can mean the house gets cold.
- *Animals*. Cat dander can be avoided by not keeping a cat, or disposing of the existing one – but some people like cats and find that the quality of their lives is reduced if they do not have one. In fact, there is evidence that in older people who live alone the presence of a pet reduces loneliness, thereby reducing physical disease because of improved immune system functioning.
- *Cigarette smoke*. This can be avoided if the patient avoids public places where smoking is allowed – but some people like going to pubs, clubs and other places where smoking is allowed. Some patients smoke, and smoking is an addiction which is very hard to break.
- *Food sensitivity*. If patients are sensitive to foods then avoidance of those foods can improve PEF. However, dietary restrictions are an inconvenience.

In cases like those above, it is best to present avoidance as an option, and discuss with the patient what overall is the best strategy for maintaining a good quality of life. In some cases (e.g., feather pillows) there may be little quality-of-life loss from avoidance. In the case of others (e.g., cats) the patient may prefer to suffer rather than avoid the trigger situation. Different patients will opt for patterns of avoidance or tolerance of triggers: some will dispose of the cat; others will not.

Box 4.11 Reducing dander in animals

Cat and other animal dander can be reduced by regular washing. Although some animals do not seem enthusiastic about being washed, even a wash once per week can be of some help.

If triggers are difficult to avoid, then the triggers can be managed to some extent by anticipatory medication, and the use of medicine in this way will also contribute to a sense of control over asthma. Exercise-induced asthma can be managed by a β-agonist before the exercise. If the patient is going on holiday, then inhaled steroid dose can be doubled during the period of the holiday. Similarly, if the patient is going to a party, then inhaled steroid dose can be increased for a couple of days before going. Some triggers are more difficult to manage, and these include psychological triggers such as stress, and the trigger occurring in women of being premenstrual – a trigger which may either be psychological or biological in nature.

CONCLUSIONS

A self-management plan is a set of 'if–then' instructions negotiated in the context of asthma education. Because patients differ both physiologically and psychologically, a single self-management plan is unlikely to be the optimum for all patients. In terms of psychological variation, plans need to accommodate two extreme types of patient. At one end is the patient who says 'tell me what to do, and I want it to be simple; I just don't want to find out. You are the expert you tell me'. At the other end is the patient who says 'It's my body and I need to be convinced that what I am doing is right for me. Tell me what you know and I will make up my own mind about what is best for me'. Most patients fall somewhere in between those two extremes, and are managed best by a plan appropriate to the level of the patient's desire for control self-determination.

REFERENCES

Abramson L Y, Seligman M E P, Teasdale J D 1978 Learned helplessness in humans: Critique and reformulation. Journal of Abnormal Psychology 87: 49–74

Baddeley A 1996 Human memory: theory and practice. Erlbaum, London

Beasley R, Cushley M, Holgate S T 1989 A self management plan in the treatment of adult asthma. Thorax 44: 200–204

Deci E L, Ryan R M 1985 Intrinsic motivation and self-determination in human behaviour. Plenum Press, New York

Frankenhauser M 1986 A psychobiological framework for research on human stress and coping. In: Appley M H, Trumbull R (eds) Dynamics of stress: physiological, psychological and social perspectives. Plenum, New York, pp. 101–116

Hyland M E 1988 Motivational control theory: an integrative framework. Journal of Personality and Social Psychology 55: 642–651

Hyland M E 1997 How do patients operate self-management plans? Asthma in General Practice 4: 12–14

International Consensus Report on Diagnosis and Treatment of Asthma 1992 National Institutes of Health (Publication No. 92–3091), Bethesda, MD

Janis I L, Feshback S 1953 Effects of fear-arousing communications. Journal of Abnormal and Social Psychology 48: 78–92

Klingelhofer E L, Gershwin M E 1988 Asthma self-management programs: premises, not promises. Journal of Asthma 25: 89–101

Raps C C, Peterson C, Jonas M, Seligman M E P 1982 Patient behaviour in hospitals: helplessness, reactance, or both? Journal of Personality and Social Psychology 42: 1036–1041

Rodin J, Langer E J 1977 Long-term effects of a control-relevant intervention with the institutionalized aged. Journal of Personality and Social Psychology 35: 897–902

Seligman M E P 1975 Helplessness: on depression, development and death. Freeman, San Francisco

Sieber W J, Rodin J, Larson L et al 1992 Modulation of human natural killer cell activity by exposure to uncontrollable stress. Brain, Behavior, and Immunity 6: 1–16

White R W 1959 Motivation reconsidered: the concept of competence. Psychological Review 66: 319–327

Winefield A H 1983 Cognitive performance deficits induced by exposure to response-independent positive outcomes. Motivation and Emotion 7: 185–195

Changing and individualising self-management plans so as to improve quality of life

5

CONTENTS

There are occasions when self-management plans need to be changed or refined in some way, either because of physiological changes or because of psychological changes. These adjustments to self-management plans are necessary to maximise quality of life over the longer term. This chapter covers how adjustments to self-management plans can be tailored to the needs of individual patients, and covers both assessments and possible change alternatives.

LONG-TERM PERSPECTIVE ON QUALITY OF LIFE

If people are asked to name the different parts of their life that contribute to their 'quality of life', they name many things, including family, friends, work, religion – and health. Health is one of several things that can contribute to quality of life, but it is not the only thing, and for some people it isn't very important (McGee et al 1991). Health is one of those things you notice when you haven't got it. It tends to become more important as health deteriorates, but, for healthy people, family or pleasure may be seen as more important contributors to quality of life. Health is important once you lose it!

This observation is important when one compares people with and without asthma. If the overall aim is to improve the total quality of life of the patient then one should not only try to control asthma, but also to reduce the extent to which controlling asthma is perceived as a health burden. The aim is to control asthma but leave people feeling 'normal' and 'well', so that asthma care is minimal and patients can get on with the other things in their lives.

A useful analogy is the way people feel about brushing their teeth. The majority of the population brush their teeth morning and evening. Everyone knows that brushing of teeth is preventive of dental decay. But people do not feel that they must have 'bad teeth' when they brush them. Nor does brushing teeth remind people that their teeth may fall out when they get old. Brushing of teeth is done automatically; it does not impose a health burden, and it does not give the message 'you are an unhealthy person'. I have never heard anyone saying 'Oh, if only I didn't have to brush my teeth every day, wouldn't life be grand'. But many people with asthma would much rather not have to take their inhaler twice per day.

In developing self-management plans over the longer term, the health professional needs to prevent the self-management plan in itself becoming a burden. Good quality of life needs more than good asthma control; it also needs a nondisruptive self-management plan.

CHANGING DRUGS AND DEVICES

Overview of treatment change options

Just as patients have 'action points' when they change their pattern of drug use, so health professionals have action points when they need to change the self-management plan of the patient. The actions of change include:

- stepping up or stepping down the level of drug treatment according to the BTS sequence of treatment steps (see Ch. 1)
- changing treatment within a step, including changing drugs or devices.

Changing the patient's treatment depends on evidence of good or poor control. However, it is important to emphasise that stepping up treatment (i.e., shifting to a higher step in the BTS guidelines) should be considered only when issues of compliance have been ruled out (see Ch. 6). Specifically, a step up in treatment should be considered only if:

- the patient is taking the correct amount of drug
- the patient is using the device correctly.

Criteria for good and poor control

The British Thoracic Society Guidelines (British Thoracic Society 1993, British Asthma Guidelines Coordinating Committee 1997) suggest that the meaning of *good control* at Steps 1–3 is different to the meaning of *good control* at Steps 4 and 5. To summarise, patients at Steps 1–3 should have little physiological or quality-of-life abnormality, whereas those at Steps 4 and 5 have as little abnormality as possible. Good control is defined in terms of five outcomes: PEF, symptoms, relief bronchodilators, quality of life, and drug side effects.

• *PEF*. Asthma control is good if daily PEF values are typically greater or equal to about 80% of best and there is a difference in morning and evening PEF values of less than 20%. Poor asthma control occurs if either of these targets is not met.

• *Symptom reporting*. The BTS guidelines use the term 'minimal symptoms' as the aim of treatment, though exactly how minimal is *minimal* is not defined. A common interpretation is that symptoms should be occurring less than once per day, for Step 3 and below. At Steps 4 and 5 the aim is to have as few symptoms as possible.

- *Relief bronchodilator use*. Again, the BTS guidelines use the term 'minimal' in relation to use. Relief bronchodilator use is strongly associated with symptom reporting, and so the BTS definition of 'minimal use' can also be interpreted as less than once per day for Step 3 and below. The North of England evidence-based guidelines (North of England Asthma Guideline Development Group 1996) make this specific, saying 'Increase treatment if using β agonist two or three doses daily *or poor control*' (italics added).
- *Quality of life*. The BTS guidelines refer to activity restriction in particular in relation to exercise, and suggest that if there is good control then there should be no limitation.
- *Drug side effect*. The aim is to have no or minimal side effects. Minimal side effects are difficult to quantify, but, for example, one could infer occasions of oral *Candida* of less than twice per year.

Deciding about control

In some instances, recognition of 'good control' and 'poor control' is straightforward. If the patient meets all the above criteria then the patient is 'well controlled'. Similarly, if the patient wakes frequently at night because of asthma, has diurnal variation of about 30% and is using relief medication ten times a day, then the patient is 'poorly controlled'. But what about the patient with good PEF who is waking once a fortnight with symptoms, or once a week, or slightly more than once a week, or twice a week? What happens if patients are out of control on one indicator but not on any of the others?

In practice, level of control varies continuously between good control and poor control. In the middle, between good and poor control, there is a kind of indeterminate range where different experts will not always agree about whether control has been achieved or not. It is therefore useful to think about this indeterminate range in terms of the objectives of maintaining asthma control.

First, consider the case of a patient A who has PEF variability of about 10%, no history of exacerbations (i.e., no unscheduled visits, and no report of asthma attacks), but who reports having minor symptoms at least once per day, and doesn't like using a bronchodilator. Patient A is just within the guideline criteria for poor control on just one of the criteria, namely, symptoms, but not, note, relief bronchodilators.

Compare patient A with patient B who has PEF variability of 25%, exacerbations about once or twice per year, but no symptoms. Patient B is just within the guideline criteria for poor control on just one of the criteria, namely, PEF.

One view is that both patients require treatment because they both fail all the criteria of good control specified in the BTS guidelines. An alternative view is that if patient A is not bothered by the symptoms, and patient B's exacerbations are not at all serious, then increased therapy is not needed. Either view may be supported depending on the precise characteristics of the patient, but in trying to make a decision one should consider two primary objectives of asthma management:

1. The management should be conservative to avoid any possible risk of fatality. The question to be asked, therefore, in considering change, is 'How safe is the patient?'.

2. The management should try to improve the quality of life of the patient as defined by the patient. The question to be asked is 'What are the consequences for quality of life of changing or not changing treatment?'.

In order to come to a decision about asthma control for patients in the indeterminate range, one needs to know not only the criteria specified in the BTS guidelines, but also other information about the patient, information relating to the level of risk and preference for lifestyle. For example, if patient A, in the example above, is an athlete for whom symptoms are a major problem, then the health professional should be much more ready to consider patient A to be poorly controlled than if patient A were someone for whom physical activity was unimportant. In addition to patient preference, the health professional should take risk into account. How safe has the patient been in the past? Is there any change taking place? What is the patient's compliance like? If the patient has a history of risk, the health professional should be more ready to move up a step. Borderline cases of control, such as those described above, can be resolved by taking into account additional information to that specified in the guidelines.

When coming to a decision in apparently borderline cases, as well as some not so borderline cases, one should always consider the possibility that patients are not fully aware of the benefits of modern asthma treatments. Due to psychological adaptation to asthma (i.e., disengagement), some patients may be unaware that improvement is possible. For such patients it may be helpful to suggest a trial period with a change in medication, with a fixed time for review.

Box 5.1 Example of patient underestimation of effect of asthma on quality of life

Q: Does asthma disturb you at night?

A: Oh no.

Q: How often do you get woken at night because of your asthma?

A: About once, very occasionally twice.

Q: Isn't that a case of asthma disturbing your sleep?

A: No, not really. I mean it's normal. Asthma only disturbs my sleep if I can't get back to sleep again.

As noted in Chapter 3, some patients are inclined not to complain about quality-of-life problems, perhaps because they have developed avoidance strategies for problems. Thus, optimistic, noncomplaining patients may lose out simply because of their way of interacting with health professionals. My guess is that patients who show particular concern about the health professional's wellbeing are prone to underestimate their own problems, so it might be worth being particularly vigilant with patients who ask about your own health and feelings.

Actions on detecting good or poor asthma control

Good control

For patients whose asthma control is good, there is often little required. The only question which needs to be answered is, 'Is the patient overmedicated at the present step?' The answer to this question can be discovered from a trial period at a reduced level of medication, but such trials do not have to be carried out at all frequently. Asthma morbidity can reduce spontaneously, though such occurrences are uncommon in the adult population.

Nevertheless it is certainly worth reviewing well-controlled patients on an annual basis and, for those where control is excellent and there is the possibility of overmedication, then a trial of reduced dosage should be instigated. Such trials, however, do need careful monitoring, and should be considered only after 3 to 6 months of stability – with allowances made for seasonal exacerbations of asthma.

Stepping down should be done slowly, and the BTS guidelines suggest that inhaled steroids should be reduced by between 25% and 50% with a 1 to 3 month interval between steps. The reason why stepping down should be slow is that, if there is going to be an increase in inflammation after step down, it is difficult to predict how soon that increase will occur, as the rate of increase differs between patients. For some patients, a reduction in steroid produces increased inflammation and reduced PEF after a matter of days. You will therefore know whether step down is possible very soon. For other patients, however, the inflammatory cycle only starts emerging after a matter of months, so that deterioration appears only at about 3 months after step down. My own suggestion is that patients need fairly careful monitoring for a year after step down, to allow for seasonal variation. Nevertheless, the BTS guidelines make the point that stepping is often not adequately attended to, at least by health professionals – patients can be more enthusiastic about stepping down; see the next chapter on compliance.

Poor control

The more complex case arises where the patient is poorly controlled. Several factors need then to be considered. First, does the patient comply with treatment – i.e., takes the prescribed dose of anti-inflammatory medicine? If so, is the patient using the device correctly? If both of these can be answered in the affirmative, then can a change of device or drug *at the same step* resolve the problem? Alternatively, should an increase in step be considered?

The important point to emphasise is that although an increase in step in treatment is often called for when poor control is detected, an increase in step is not the only option that should be considered. There is considerably more patient specificity in response to asthma treatments than may be apparent from the recommendations of drug companies – as well as published clinical trials. In addition, the device can make a substantial difference. Sometimes budesonide works better than beclomethasone or vice versa. Sometimes generic salbutamol does not work as well as Ventolin – possibly due to differences in droplet size produced by different MDIs but possibly also for psychological reasons. What works for one patient may not work for another, and so the best way of optimising drug treatments is to try a particular therapy and monitor the result.

Box 5.2 Case study

Mr Jones is poorly controlled on Step 2 and is currently prescribed 400 μg beclomethasone via an MDI (i.e., standard dose inhaled steroid). Mr Jones takes his inhaled steroid regularly as indicated by clinic records of repeat prescriptions. The recommended course of action is to increase medication to Step 3. Two options are possible at Step 3: first, changing to high-dose inhaled steroid; second, changing to standard-dose inhaled steroid plus long-acting bronchodilator. The health professional tries the first option in the first instance, but Mr Jones reports no improvement. Mr Jones is then switched to the standard-dose inhaled steroid plus long-acting bronchodilator, and Mr Jones improves substantially. The health professional reasoned that if Mr Jones reported no benefits from the high-dose inhaled steroid, then he was probably achieving a ceiling effect, despite only being on low-dose inhaled steroid. Other options open to the health professional would have been to change the type of steroid once the high-dose beclomethasone proved unsatisfactory (i.e., change to 800 μg budesonide or 400 μg fluticasone) or to add another anti-inflammatory medicine to the standard-dose inhaled steroid, for example, adding on an anti-leukotriene to the 400 μg of beclomethasone.

Device selection

Familiarity

Inhaled medicines are normally provided by two types of device: metered dose inhalers (MDIs), and dry powder inhalers. However, to the patient, the device is not just an object that delivers medicine. It is an object which has certain familiarity, ease of use, and aesthetic appeal. Just as people have favourite clothes, and just as gardeners often have a favourite pair of secateurs or garden fork, so people with asthma develop preferences for inhalers. And like clothes and garden secateurs, different people like different things. If a patient feels comfortable with a particular device, then that feeling of comfort is in itself a contributor to asthma quality of life. As a general rule, patients tend to like the device they are familiar with (or devices similar to the one they are familiar with), and so patients will often be conservative in change.

Ease of operation

Devices vary in their ease of operation in several ways, and what is easy to use for one patient may not be easy to use for another. Lack of coordination between actuation and inhalation is a major problem with standard MDIs, and this problem is not present in the case of dry powder inhalers, breath-actuated MDIs or standard MDIs with a spacer. Spacers vary in size, but the large ones are much more effective than the small ones. However, large spacers are difficult to carry around and have a greater stigmatising effect than a small inhaler. Some patients discontinue using a spacer even if recommended.

Some devices require more manual dexterity than others. Dry powder inhalers can, in some cases, be fiddly to reload. Older people with clumsy fingers and people with large fingers may find devices difficult to use that others find easy. Whether or not two hands are needed, whether or not it is necessary to look before operating (i.e., requiring reasonable light levels or good eyesight) are all factors which affect ease of use.

Some dry powder inhalers deteriorate if kept in a bathroom, so a problem may arise if the patient has a routine of taking medicine at the same time as brushing teeth.

Some patients are unable to stop the back of the mouth closing when using a standard MDI, because of the effect of the cold inhalant being sprayed into the mouth, though a new form of MDI helps to prevent this problem by ensuring that the spray comes out at a much slower speed. This new low-velocity aerosol has a small built-in spacer which is as effective as a standard MDI with large inhaler.

Feedback

Two kinds of feedback are useful to the patient: feedback about how many doses are left, and feedback about whether a dose has been taken correctly. It is possible to judge whether an MDI is getting empty by floating it in water, but this is such a bother that few patients will do it. More recent devices have counters which count down the number of available doses or indicate when a new inhaler is needed. Some new MDIs and reservoir-based dry powder inhalers have a 'lock out' facility so the patient cannot use the inhaler when no drug is left.

Feedback about whether a dose has been taken correctly is also helpful. In some cases, patients obtain feedback from taste. One dry powder device has a whistle which can be added to show whether inspiration is sufficiently fast. Newer devices have feedback windows showing adequacy of use.

Technical properties of inhaler and interaction with technique

The amount of drug delivered to the lungs by both MDIs and drug powder inhalers depends on the device, and some devices are considerably better in this regard than others. In addition, the amount of drug delivered to the lungs depends on technique. Some dry powder inhalers require a reasonable level of inspiration to create a good dispersion of drug in air. However, too fast an inspiration in an MDI can lead to particles being deposited on the back of the throat. As a general rule, breathing should not be too rapid with an MDI, nor too slow with a dry powder device. In the case of dry powder devices, the amount of drug getting into the lungs increases with rate of inspiration (some inhalers are more sensitive to this effect than others), so if the inhaler has a high degree of inspiratory resistance and the patient is weak, then the device may not be optimal for drug delivery. One should be aware that two patients who have identical prescriptions may be receiving different doses of drug. The technical properties of the inhaler interact with technique.

Box 5.3 Case study

Mrs Webster could not use an MDI, because of difficulty of coordination, but used it successfully with a large-volume spacer. Mrs Webster was going on holiday for a week shortly, and casually mentioned to the asthma nurse that she wasn't going to take her brown inhaler – because the spacer was too cumbersome to pack in her suitcase. The asthma nurse provided a dry powder inhaler for the holiday, and made a mental note to check about holidays for all patients who used a spacer!

Patient preference

Research on patient preferences for devices shows there to be substantial differences in preference. Just as people like different types of breakfast cereal, so patients have their own particular preference for type of device. Particular devices are often associated with particular drugs, so device selection by patients needs to be incorporated into the more general aim of ensuring optimal drug treatment.

If you were buying a new car, you would to be able to look at the range of cars available in your price range, and to try out the ones which you were interested in. In order to make an informed choice, the patient should see different devices, and try them out, before making a decision. Patients may also need a little time to make up their minds – people can take a while to decide which car to buy. If patients have difficulty choosing, they should be given the opportunity to try different inhalers at home, rather than necessarily having to choose in the clinic.

The reason for giving choice is not simply a matter of pandering to patients' aesthetic whims. Choice provides a sense of control and involvement. Choice encourages compliance because the patient feels that he or she has chosen the medicine, rather than being subjected to an imposed regimen. Choice of device is particularly important for patients with a high need for control, who believe their health depends on their own actions, and who take a problem-focused approach to coping.

However, as there are so many devices available and coming onto the market, it is not possible or practical to give all patients complete choice. In addition, some patients, those with a low need for control, may want one to be given rather than to exert a choice. A useful strategy is for health professionals involved in asthma care to decide on a range of inhalers that can be offered to patients, and allow patients to choose from that range. It may be possible to have different ranges for different types of patients. Although patient choice is important, the health professional will still act as a gatekeeper to that choice.

Other factors affecting choice

Two other factors affect choice of device: the side effects and the cost of the device to the practice. The topic of side effects is important in its own right, and is discussed in the next section. If drug budgets are limited, as they invariably are, then devices may be chosen on the basis of cost, and issues of rationing will be covered in Chapter 7.

Box 5.4 Features to consider when selecting a device

- What does the patient want?
  - perceived convenience?
  - aesthetic appeal to patient?
  - is it discrete?
  - is it the right 'image' for the patient?
  - can it be carried around easily?
  - is it easy to use?
  - does inhalation make the patient cough?
  - does it taste unpleasant?
- Can the patient use it effectively?
  - ease of coordination?
  - ease of inspiration?
  - ease of reloading?
  - is it easy to keep clean?
- Does the device give feedback?
  - counters indicating when a new one is needed?
  - indicator as to whether the dose is taken correctly?
  - counters indicating whether dose taken today?
- Is the dose consistent over the life of the device?
  - does dose become erratic when becoming empty?
  - does the patient need to puff into the air to ensure correct dose when device not used recently?
- How much of the drug gets into the lungs and how much elsewhere?
  - particle size, respirable fraction?
  - side effect profile when using device?
- Is it expensive? (Note: newer devices tend to be better and also more expensive)
  - cost per actuation to health centre?
  - cost per actuation to patient?

Side effects

One of the criteria of good control in the BTS guidelines is the absence of, or the presence of only minimal, side effects. Side effects vary substantially between patients – some get side effects and some do not, in a way which is relatively unpredictable. Side effects also depend on dose and mode of delivery. Oral steroids produce much greater side effects than inhaled steroids, and high-dose inhaled more than low-dose inhaled. The following comments apply to steroids unless stated otherwise.

Types of side effect

There are two classes of side effects: local and systemic. Local side effects are associated only with inhaled delivery and occur at the site of drug administration, i.e., the mouth and throat. Local side effects consist of oral *Candida* (a fungal infection), sore throat (viral or bacterial), and hoarseness. Systemic side effects are found with both inhaled and oral delivery and occur at other sites throughout the body. Systemic effects include (but are not limited to) adrenal suppression, bone density changes, skin thinning leading to easy bruising, and possibly greater proneness to infection – steroids have an immunosuppressant effect.

Side effects from standard-dose inhaled steroids are rare and limited to local effects. The side effects of high-dose inhaled steroids are less rare, though still uncommon, and include local effects as well as systemic effects. Oral steroids when used regularly do not have any of the local effects, but they do have systemic effects which are more serious. In addition to those listed above, regular use of inhaled steroids leads to weight gain and a puffy 'cushingoid' appearance which some patients find very distressing, as well as a variety of other physiological changes. Patients prescribed regular steroids should be referred to a respiratory consultant. Some patients need courses of oral steroids as rescue therapy, and it is believed that systemic effects are unlikely if no more than three 10 day courses of oral steroids are prescribed per year. In addition, to considering side effects, the effects of tolerance should also be considered in relation to drug use. Tolerance effects refer to the possibility that a drug is less effective after a period of use compared with when it is first used.

As a rule of thumb, standard doses of inhaled steroids are safe, and the likelihood of side effects is extremely low. High-dose inhaled steroids can produce side effects. Regular oral steroids do produce side effects. Occasional use of oral steroids produces side effects only if more than three courses are needed in a year. In all cases, however, there are actions that can reduce the frequency or extent of side effects, and seven courses of action are described below.

Minimising local effects

Minimisation of local effects can be achieved by ensuring that the inhaled particles get into the lungs rather than being deposited in the throat and mouth. The following three actions all achieve this effect

1. MDIs and dry powder inhalers vary considerably in the way they deposit drugs in the lung. As a general rule, the newer devices of both kinds are much more efficient than older devices. For example, the non-CFC inhalers (HFAs) provide a much better dispersion of beclomethasone than the standard MDIs, and the newer powder inhalers are also slightly better than the standard MDIs. Changing to a more recent device can reduce the likelihood of local side effects. The health professional should ask manufacturers for details about deposition of the drug in the lung (bronchi and bronchioles), throat and alveoli. Note that this calculation depends very much on the method employed, so the manufacturer's data should be treated with caution. For example, there is normally better deposition of the drug in healthy volunteers than in people with asthma. The amount deposited also depends on the technique of the patient.

2. An MDI produces particles of varying sizes. The large particles tend to get stuck in the mouth, whereas the small particles are able to travel into the lungs. If a spacer is used between the MDI and mouth, then the larger particles stick to the side of the spacer, leaving the small particles to travel into the lung. Small spacers are less effective in this regard, so the disadvantage of using a spacer is that, the more effective ones are quite large (see Box 5.3). Spacers should be air dried rather than rubbed dry, as rubbing creates an electrostatic charge which reduces their ability to attract the large particles. Improved design of a recent low-velocity MDI which has its own built-in small spacer, however, makes it as efficient as a standard MDI plus large spacer (though it is more expensive).

3. If patients wash their mouths out after inhaling (brushing of teeth and gargling can also be included) then a good deal of drug deposited in the mouth will be washed out.

The above points should be considered for patients even if they are not experiencing side effects, but, of course, spacers and mouth washing provide additional bother which detracts from quality of life. However, for patients who are anxious about the effect of steroids, the ability to do something about it, something which is the patient's responsibility, can help reduce this anxiety.

Systemic effects of steroids

Systemic effects result from inhaled steroids entering the blood stream or from oral steroids which have a mode of action via the blood stream. Inhaled medicines enter the circulatory system through two routes: through the lungs, and through the deposited particles in the throat being swallowed into the stomach. When entering the lungs, small amounts of the inhaled steroid enter the circulatory system, where they are widely dispersed throughout the body. When entering through the stomach – which tends to be the case for most of the inhaled drug – the drug passes initially through the liver before entering the general circulation.

4. Different types of inhaled steroid have different side effect profiles. Any action which reduces local side effects will also reduce systemic entry through the stomach/liver route. Hence actions 1–3 should all be considered, and the MDI with a large-volume spacer will again be the safest type of device. But there is an additional consideration, and that is that some types of steroid are broken down in the liver, so that the effect of the stomach/liver route is abolished or at least substantially reduced for those steroids. The 'first generation' steroid, beclomethasone, is broken down only moderately in the liver, whereas the 'second generation' steroids, budesonide and fluticasone, are broken down to a much greater extent. Hence the side effect profile of the second-generation steroids is safer than that of beclomethasone, and this may be a consideration for patients on high-dose steroids, particularly those on very high doses. However, it should be stressed that systemic effects are normally only noticeable, and only in some cases, with high-dose inhaled steroids.

Box 5.5 Optimising delivery of inhaled drugs

New devices are designed to ensure that the drug enters the lungs rather than being deposited in the back of the throat. Small particles tend to get down into the lungs, whereas the larger particles get deposited in the throat. Recently, there has been increased attention to ensuring that the particles get to the right place in the lungs. The very smallest particles are deposited in the alveoli where they are quickly absorbed into the blood stream without having any beneficial effect. It may be that the best areas for deposition of steroids differ from the best areas for deposition of bronchodilators – research is still being done.

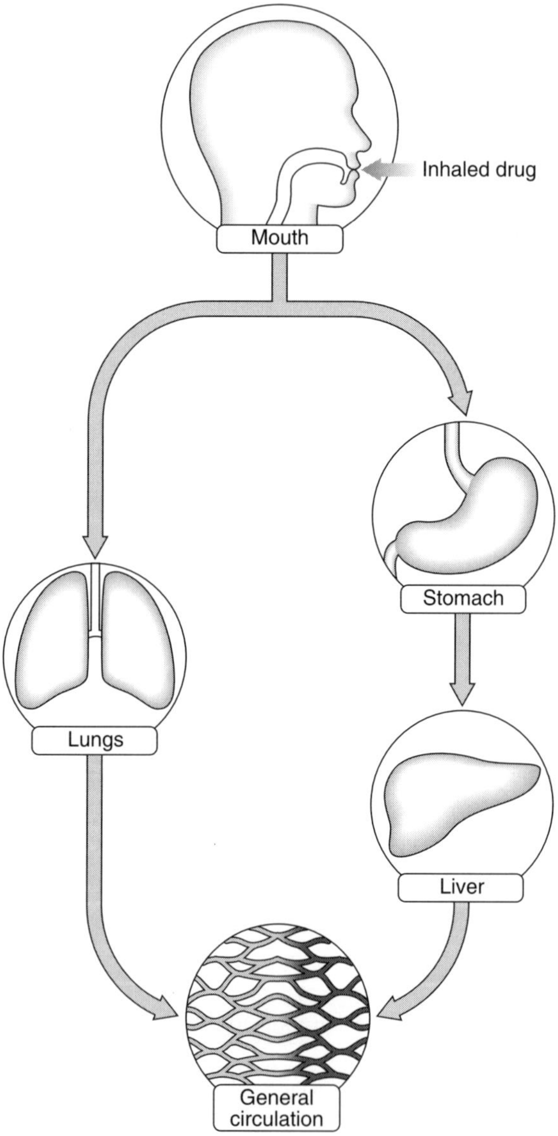

Fig. 5.1 Two routes of steroid systemic entry.

A patient may have side effects with one type of steroid but not with another. Hence shifting patients from one steroid to another, or from one steroid–device combination to another is an option to consider if side effects cause problems.

There is an additional factor which needs to considered, particularly with regard to patient preference of devices. The newer devices, both MDIs and dry powder, have a better side effect profile than the earlier equivalents. However, this advantage is much less important when the second-generation steroids are used. The reason is that the systemic consequence of deposition in the mouth is very much less with the second-generation steroids, as these are broken down in the liver. Local effects, however, still remain more likely with older devices

5. Side effects may be reduced by changing types of drugs within the same step. In addition to changing the type of steroid or device, another option is available for patients on high-dose steroid at Step 3. You will recall that at Step 3 there are two treatment options: strong anti-inflammatory, or mild anti-inflammatory plus long acting bronchodilator. If patients are experiencing side effects on high-dose steroid, then an alternative treatment option would be low-dose steroid plus long-acting β-agonist. Note: combined inhaled steroid plus long-acting β-agonist inhalers reduce the burden of inhaler use on the patient – and may reduce cost to the patient. In the future, when anti-leukotrienes are more developed, another option may be low-dose steroid plus anti-leukotriene.

It is much more difficult to manage side effects in the case of oral steroids. When a patient is prescribed oral steroids, it is important to stress that this is unwanted but unavoidable treatment, because the health risk of not having the steroid is greater than the risk of having it. Side effects can be reduced to some extent by timing the administration of the steroid to coincide with the body's natural rhythm of corticosteroid production, namely in the mid to early morning. The side effect profile of oral steroids depends on dose and on the half-life of the drug. Prednisolone is used in asthma because it has a relatively short half-life compared with other steroids, and therefore has lower systemic effects.

6. Patients should be encouraged to adopt lifestyles which ameliorate the effects of steroids on bone. One of the systemic effects of steroids, which is particularly important to older women, is the tendency for calcium to be leached out of bone, leading to bones which are brittle and fracture easily. Bone chemistry and strength is, however, affected by many other factors, including diet and exercise. A diet rich in calcium, in particular dairy products and tinned fish, helps maintain bones in good condition – in fact it is the bones in the

tinned fish that are high in calcium, so patients should ensure they eat the bones in tinned sardines and salmon. Bones are also very much affected by exercise – in particular, exercise which puts a load-bearing strain on the bone. Although we should not expect patients to take up weight lifting, any form of exercise or leisure activity that requires strength will be good.

7. Patients should be encouraged to adopt healthy lifestyles. All steroids, both produced naturally and taken as medicine, suppress the immune system, either at the point of drug action or, if absorbed in the blood stream, systemically. The immune system is affected by a variety of other factors, both psychological and physiological, some of which may be under the patient's control. In particular, lack of exercise, high (but socially acceptable) intake of alcohol, and high intake of sugary foods can act as immunosuppressants, as does emotional upset and depression. If patients experience local side effects associated with infection, it is worth exploring the possibility of improving immunocompetence through lifestyle.

Side effects of other drugs

β-agonists can cause tremor (usually in the hands), a racing heart, a feeling of tension or nervousness, and headaches. The likelihood of these effects depends on dose, and none will be serious even with the high dose of bronchodilators administered in an asthma attack. There are rare cases where β-agonists cause a paradoxical bronchospasm Theophylline causes racing heart, as well as nausea and stomach upset. The effects are dose dependent, and in contrast to β-agonists, overdosing has serious adverse consequences. Cromoglycate has no side effects other than the coughing from the irritation of inhalation; in addition to the coughing, nedocromil can (rarely) cause headache, nausea and vomiting. The side effects of anti-leukotrienes are not established as yet.

Tolerance and withdrawal effects

There is no evidence of tolerance effects with regard to steroids; that is, the steroid is as effective at the beginning as at the end of a course of treatment. The removal of inhaled steroids does not produce withdrawal problems. However, the removal of regular oral steroids does cause withdrawal problems, and such withdrawal should be slow. By contrast, there are no withdrawal problems for short rescue courses of oral steroids, because adrenal suppression has not occurred to any degree. Hence short courses of oral steroids do not need tapering down.

There has been some concern about the possibility of tolerance effects with respect to β-agonists, but there is lack of consensus on this point. The possibility has been raised that continuous use of β-agonists results in this drug's being less effective in an asthma attack. Although there is no clear support for this view, either for short-acting or long-acting β-agonists, the possibility of tolerance with β-agonists has been used to uphold the view that control of inflammation is the primary aim of asthma management.

Sequencing of drugs and devices

At any step in the BTS guidelines, the health professional is faced with a wide choice of drugs and devices. Sequencing refers to the order in which different treatments are given to the patient as part of a therapeutic trial carried out to see whether a particular treatment is effective or not. Of course, sequencing must be kept in perspective. Although some patients respond better to some drugs and to some devices, the majority of patients usually respond well to any of the available steroids. Therapeutic trials of one drug or another are neither practical nor needed in all patients. The question of sequencing of drugs on a therapeutic trial is most likely to arise with nonsteroidal 'add ons' to prophylactic therapy at Step 3 and above. For example, the BTS guidelines at Step 4 suggest that the patient should have high-dose steroid (800–2000 μg daily of either beclomethasone or budesonide via MDI plus spacer, or 400–1000 μg fluticasone) plus a sequential trial of the following:

- inhaled long-acting β-agonist
- sustained-release theophylline
- inhaled ipratoprium or oxitropium
- long-acting β-agonist tablets
- high-dose inhaled bronchodilators
- cromoglycate or nedocromil.

In practical terms, this means the health professional tries the drug at the top of the list, and, if that doesn't work, stops that drug and tries the drug next down the list (about 1 to 2 weeks is sufficient for a trial). Note that if the first drug is not effective, then it is discontinued, but if a drug is to some extent effective, then this does not exclude the use of other drugs in combination.

The sequence recommended by the BTS is based on a mixture of an understanding of disease processes and clinical experience, but really there is no scientific basis for one sequence versus another. Sequencing is needed because one cannot predict in advance what treatment is going to be most effective in an individual case. Indeed, for many treatments the *average* effects of treatments over large groups of patients are rather similar.

Although pharmaceutical representatives provide evidence for the superiority of their own products, it is worth considering the comments from an evidence-based set of guidelines (North of England Asthma Guideline Development Group 1996), which is based on reviews of several clinical trials. Here are some extracts from those guidelines.

> There are no clinically important differences in effectiveness between the various inhaled steroids that cannot be addressed by dosage adjustment.
>
> As there is no good evidence of clinically important differences between differing inhaled steroids, patients should be treated with the cheapest inhaled steroid they can use and which controls their symptoms.
>
> There is no evidence to prefer nedocromil to sodium cromoglycate or vice versa.

Of course, these conclusions are based on *average* response in clinical trials and should not blind one to the very real differences that occur in some patients – both in terms of efficacy and side effects. Certainly some patients respond better to some treatments than to others.

The sequencing of inhaler devices is driven more by cost, patient competence and preference than by any evidence of efficacy. The North of England guidelines comment is:

> Metered dose inhalers are as effective as powder devices, and autohalers are no more effective than metered dose inhalers.

In fact, the invention of recent devices means that this statement is less true now than it was then, but nevertheless it draws attention to the fact that, when used correctly, the different devices are all effective. However, an effective device is ineffective when used ineffectively; the crucial question, and one which should determine choice of inhaler, is not 'How effective is this inhaler?' but How effective will this inhaler be when used by this particular patient?'.

It is worth reflecting that choice when sequencing drugs should be determined mainly by preferences of the health professional, whereas choice when sequencing devices should be determined mainly by preferences of the patient.

The Step 3 alternative

Step 3 in the BTS guidelines offers an important choice: high-dose steroid versus low-dose steroid plus long acting β-agonist. This is an important difference, and it is worth taking a moment to reflect on how the health professional should handle this choice. The choice is thought to arise because the dose response curve varies between patients (see Fig. 5.2). So, for some patients, the effectiveness of the steroid ceases to increase at doses of about 1000 μg beclomethasone via MDI or equivalent, and a long-acting bronchodilator is added to treatment at Step 2 in the treatment. Reports from clinical experience suggest that if patients are very poorly controlled at Step 2 (for example, actual-over-best of less than 75%) then they respond better to an increase in steroids, whereas patients who experience symptoms but no serious exacerbations respond better to the long-acting bronchodilator option. As a rule of thumb, therefore, patients with poor lung function or who have a history of emergency treatment could be tried initially on the high-dose steroid option, whereas the

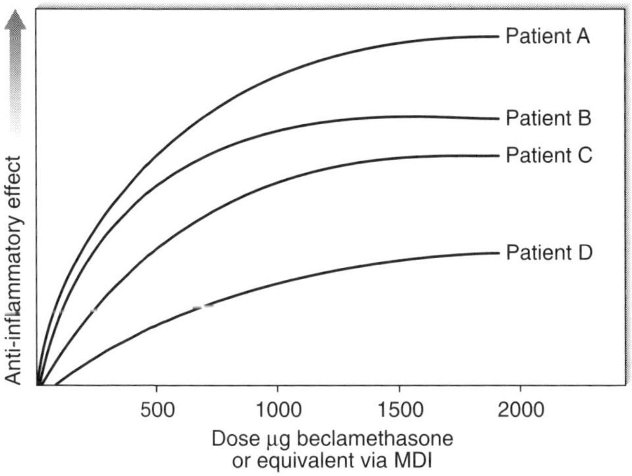

Fig. 5.2 Steroid dose response curve varies between patients.

long-acting bronchodilator option should be considered only for those patients who have comparatively better control. If there is uncontrolled inflammation, then it really does need to be treated.

DETERMINING THE ACTION POINTS IN THE SELF-MANAGEMENT PLAN

PEF versus symptoms

Self-management plans have *action points*. An action point is an event identified by the health professional for the patient to change medication or seek assistance. Action points require self-monitoring, and self-monitoring is an essential part of self-management plans, irrespective of the level of control given to the patient. In the majority of plans, patients need to know the point at which to increase prophylactic medication when asthma worsens, as a way of preventing an asthma attack. Even if the plan provides the patient with little control over dosage, the patient will need to know when to contact the doctor. What kind of self-monitoring is needed? One possible response is that patients should measure their PEF every day, preferably morning and evening, and increase their prophylactic medicine when, say 80% of best. This view was certainly held several years ago, and was a motivating force in the successful drive to enable PEF meters to be prescribed on the NHS. However, several studies have examined the effect of regular PEF monitoring on quality of life and other outcomes, and the results were surprisingly disappointing. There is no clear evidence that regular monitoring of PEF improves asthma control (Jones et al 1995). Why is this, and what consequently should health professionals recommend?

The aim of any form of self-monitoring is to predict exacerbations and so act in advance to prevent those exacerbations from occurring. PEF measurement is carried out not for its own sake but because PEF predicts asthma exacerbations. Research shows that, on average, exacerbations are much more likely to occur in the following 12 h if PEF is low: PEF is indeed a predictor of exacerbations. However, PEF is not the only predictor of exacerbations. In his observation of the early use of PEF meters, Creer (in press) found that there were three sorts of patients.

First, there are patients who learn to predict their PEF on the basis of sensations from their lungs. After an initial learning period using their PEF meter, these patients can predict PEF from their symptoms, and the PEF meter provides little additional information than is provided by their symptoms. For such patients, the PEF meter provides a useful 'teaching tool', but once the patient is experienced in interpreting symptomatology, the PEF meter is not needed on a daily basis. Patients who are able to predict the PEF well should be advised to check their PEF only when their symptoms deteriorate. Used in this way, the PEF meter simply acts as a quantitative measure of symptoms which are perceived fairly accurately. The quantitative data provides an accurate basis for action point criteria, but regular use of the PEF meter is an unnecessary burden on the patient. Occasional use triggered by developing symptoms is an acceptable self-management strategy.

Second, there are a small number of patients who believe that their symptoms provide them with more information about their lungs than do PEF readings. By more information, such patients mean that PEF is actually less useful than symptomatology in anticipating attacks. There is little research on such patients but they may well be correct in what they say. The PEF meter measures obstruction in the large or upper airways, not in the small or lower airways. If, for a particular patient, increases in inflammation start in the lower airways, and *in addition* the patient is sensitive to such lower airways changes, then symptoms will actually be more useful than the PEF meter. Hence, such patients should not use their PEF meter to anticipate attacks. The poor relationship between PEF and symptoms is because PEF provides information which is less clinically relevant. Patients should be advised to manage action points only on the basis of symptoms.

Finally, there are patients who are bad at predicting the onset of an attack on the basis of symptoms, and are unable to predict PEF from their symptoms. These patients may form a surprisingly high proportion of patients (Kendrick et al 1993). For such patients the PEF meter is the only reliable method for anticipating asthma attacks, and so should be used regularly. Such patients should be advised to monitor at least once every other day, but particularly if any change in lifestyle occurs.

Apart from physiological factors, such as poorly working receptors, there are two psychological reasons why symptoms may predict neither PEF nor exacerbations. The first reason is that

Box 5.6 Patients with poor awareness of asthma effects

In an experimental study where patients who had near-fatal asthma were compared with other asthma patients, researchers (Kikuchi et al 1994) found that patients in the near-fatal asthma group had a 'blunted perception of dyspnoea' and had 'decreased chemosensitivity to hypoxia'. In brief, when patients were made hypoxic, those who had had near-fatal asthma attacks were less aware of the fact that they were hypoxic.

From the perspective of asthma management, this means that some patients simply are unaware of how bad their lungs are functioning. Recall also that some patients do not experience much distress even when experiencing a life-threatening asthma attack. Quite simply, symptoms are an extremely poor guide to lung function in some patients.

patients' estimation of symptoms is affected by psychological factors such as attention and mood. That is, the patient notices symptoms when mood is poor or when bored, but not when mood is good or when busy. Inflammation is therefore likely to increase undetected when the patient is happily occupied in a period of high activity. Second, for some patients, anxiety and breathlessness are confused. Thus, the patient feels breathless when anxious, but not breathless when not anxious, leading to the risk of undetected increases in inflammation in periods of emotional stability. Both these reasons indicate that patients are particularly at risk for failing to detect increases in inflammation when things are going well, rather than when things are going badly. When things are going well, people can be least likely to want to learn that their asthma is going badly. The

Box 5.7 Suggested use of PEF meters and symptoms in self-monitoring

1. Patients who can accurately predict PEF from symptoms can be advised: 'Measure your PEF when you develop symptoms'.

2. Patients who cannot accurately predict PEF from symptoms are of two types and depending on the type should be advised:

a. 'Don't bother with your PEF meter' – patients whose symptoms are more accurate than PEF (note: tend to be rare)

b. 'Use your PEF meter regularly' – patients whose symptoms are less accurate than PEF.

only way to manage this problem is to ensure that patients monitor their PEF regularly, i.e., to include times when the patient is feeling happy.

Although there are undoubtedly patients who fall somewhere between these three groups, the fact that there are different types of patient leads to an important conclusion: *there is no uniform way that all patients should be recommended to use their PEF meter*.

Individualising self-monitoring for individual patients

A PEF meter is only useful to the extent that it provides additional information. If it does not provide additional information, then the daily use of a PEF meter simply has the function of imposing an additional health burden on the patient. Recommending regular PEF measurement in such cases is actually counterproductive to good quality of life – though patients are unlikely to comply in any case. The essential question to establish with the patient, therefore, is how good are their symptoms at predicting exacerbations and asthma attacks?

The answer to this question can be inferred to some extent from a careful examination of the patient's history. Patients with a history of requiring emergency treatment may be poor at detecting PEF change from symptoms. In addition, patients who are newly diagnosed as being asthmatic will almost certainly need to calibrate their symptoms to PEF. For newly diagnosed patients a routine of PEF measurement and recording is almost certainly advisable, but for patients with a history of emergency treatment a number of possible causes may be involved (see Ch. 6), so advice to carry out regular monitoring may not always produce the desired results.

In addition to examining history it is possible to test whether the patient is accurate in predicting PEF, by saying for example:

> 'Let's measure your Peak Flow to see how you are doing'.
>
> *(Gives PEF meter, smiles)*
>
> 'I wonder if you can guess what it is going to be?'

The topic of conversation can then be steered towards the patient's perception of accuracy.

A single test may not provide much information, particularly if the patient has a stable PEF, but for patients who present with a more variable PEF graph, questioning them about their ability to predict

PEF can provide information about their sensitivity to lung function changes. The use of such a test can then open the way for a frank discussion with the patient about regular or other uses of the PEF meter.

If patients become adept at interpreting their lung function from symptoms, then it is often useful to present the PEF meter as an aid for deciding on the time for an 'action point'. For example,

> 'Measure your Peak Flow every day to start with, and when you are used to what is going on, measure it every week, unless you develop symptoms. If you develop symptoms, then measure to see what is going on. Then, if your PEF is below 350, double your daily dose of the preventer inhaler – that is, four puffs in the morning and four in the evening.'

(Note how this instruction makes the meaning of 'double dose' unambiguous.)

If patients present requiring emergency treatment, it can be worth finding out about the use of the PEF meter prior to the attack. However, such questions need to be phrased tactfully, because a question such as 'How were you monitoring yourself just before the attack?' can appear inquisitorial and blaming. The patient's behaviour just prior to the attack is likely to be no different from other times, so it is worth checking on normal self-monitoring patterns before focusing on the period leading up to the attack itself, with a question such as 'Did you notice anything different about your asthma recently?'

In summary, both symptoms and PEF readings can be used to determine action points for the patient. But whether one or the other is the more useful – or whether they should be used together – depends crucially on the patient. However, irrespective of what is theoretically desirable, it is necessary to ensure that the patient feels comfortable with any particular self-monitoring process, whatever is recommended. If patients feel uncomfortable with a recommendation of self-monitoring, the chances are they will soon deviate from what has been agreed. It is better for patients to follow a self-monitoring routine that is suboptimal than to be told about the optimal one and then for them to ignore it completely.

Traffic light versus individualised PEF values

The traffic light system of using a PEF meter was described in Chapter 4. In brief, the patient is provided with ranges of PEF within which certain actions are recommended. For example, the patient may be told to double inhaled steroid dose at a value which is specified for him or her (e.g., a PEF of 250) but is in fact 80% of best. It should be noted that the PEF is used as the criterion for the action point in the majority of patients, because PEF provides a quantitative measure of deterioration that can be easily communicated to the patient. Even though the patient may know what 80% of best feels like, the health professional will not be able to describe it to the patient.

Also in Chapter 4, I indicated that different guidelines have different percentage values of PEF for the action point. Different authors and bodies have recommended different values: 60% (Clark, Evans & Mellins 1992), 70% (Beasley, Cushley & Holgate 1989), 80% (British Thoracic Society 1993, British Asthma Guidelines Coordinating Committee 1997, International Consensus Report 1992) and 90% (Charlton et al 1990). When rational people provide different recommendations, albeit small differences, the likely conclusion is that there is no clear evidence for one figure over another. However, an alternative view is that no fixed percentage figure is going to be optimal for all patients. Specifically, the disadvantage of the traffic light system is that it does not take individual differences into account, with the result that patients can be either undermedicated or overmedicated (Gibson, Murree-Allen & Saltos 1995) at any, fixed traffic light point.

An alternative approach, used by Dr Tom Creer in the USA, is based on the individualised use of PEF meters. Recall that the aim of patient-initiated increases of inhaled steroids is to anticipate and so avoid exacerbations. Creer asks patients to record their PEF and also whether they have an asthma attack in the next 12 h. If, for example, a patient records a PEF value of 250 on 10 mornings, and later has an attack on 5 out of the 10 days, then the patient has a 50% chance of an asthma attack when morning PEF is 250. Once this information is known, then when the patient has a PEF value of 250 on a future occasion, the patient can make a judgement: 'Is it worth my increasing my inhaled steroid, knowing as I do that I have a one in two chance of having an asthma attack today?'. Most patients would say 'yes', but the same decision can be made when the patient has a 1 in 3, a 1 in 4, a 1 in 10, or indeed a 1 in 50 chance of having an attack. The decision to increase steroid dose is therefore closely linked to what happens to the particular patient, rather than what happens to an average patient. In addition, the patient works out his or her own judgement of 'risk' in not increasing inhaled steroids. Thus, the patient is part of the judgement process in trying to decide on the balance between unnecessary extra medicine versus asthma-related problems.

Box 5.8 Instructions for individualised PEF values

Measure morning PEF for a period of time, ideally for at least 2 months, and keep a record of attacks, symptoms and activity problems which develop during the day. For each value of PEF, count up the number of days when there was an attack (or symptom or activity problem) and the number of days when there was no attack (or symptom or activity problem). Divide the first number by the second, multiply by 100, and you have the percentage chance of having an attack (or symptom activity problem). Present the information to the patient (see, for example, Table 5.1) and discuss when an increase in inhaled steroids seems sensible.

The use of individualised PEF values provides the patient with greater information and a sense of control. This particular approach is particularly suited to patients with a high need for control, who are reasonably competent and who cope with asthma by means of problem-focused coping. The use of individualised PEF values may be less appropriate for patients with limited cognitive ability or who want to assign responsibility and control to the health professional. In addition, finding out is a bother and requires effort which not all patients will be willing to expend.

Thus, the use of individualised PEF values is appropriate for some but not all patients who use PEF values as indicators for action points in the self-management plan. It is, of course, irrelevant to patients

Table 5.1 Example of table showing risk of events at different PEF values

Event	**PEF values**			
	250	270	300	320
Symptoms	90%	80%	60%	30%
Activity problems	60%	40%	15%	0%
Asthma attack	20%	5%	0%	0%

who believe that symptoms provide a better predictor of future asthma events.

Context-specific PEF readings

Because triggers and bronchodilators affect lung function, readings of PEF can be context specific. For example, a patient may have a best PEF value of 400, but that best value is only obtained at home, not at work, where the best value is only 350. Consistent differences in best PEF are not uncommon, and their occurrence indicates that there is something exacerbating asthma in the situation where the lower PEF value is obtained. In the example above, the patient would appear to experience some form of occupational asthma, where the conditions at work are contributing to asthma exacerbation (see next section). Context-specific effects are not necessarily occupational and may arise when visiting friends, relatives, or recreational facilities. In addition, if a patient uses a bronchodilator before measuring PEF, the reverse occurs, though the principle remains the same: PEF readings are context specific.

If context-specific PEF readings are found, then action points need to be defined in terms of those different contexts. If one simply says 'increase when you obtain a reading of only X', then patients are more likely to increase steroid dose after an experience with a trigger – which may lead to unnecessary overuse of steroids – or fail to increase steroids when PEF has been measured shortly after using a bronchodilator, leading to an insufficient use of steroids.

The importance of considering the effect of context can be illustrated further with the case of occupational asthma described above, where the best PEF reading at home was 400 and at work 350. In this case, a PEF value of 300 at home would indicate poorer control than a value of 300 obtained at work. The reason is that a value of 300 at home is 75% of a best of 400 and would indicate the need to increase steroid dose (using the traffic light system, with an action point of 80%). However, a PEF value of 300 means that this value is 86% of best obtainable in the work situation, and should lead to the conclusion that the patient is adequately controlled in a situation which exacerbates asthma. Because the value of 300 at work reflects the suppression of PEF caused by that specific situation, there is no justification in increasing steroid dose. The same caution would also need to be applied to patients who use individualised PEF action points. Whatever PEF value is selected as an action point, the meaning of that value in terms of underlying inflammation is radically different in the absence of or in the presence of a transient bronchoconstrictor or bronchodilator.

In fact, the discovery of context-specific PEF readings is very useful in terms of trigger management. As already indicated, consistent lower readings at work will indicate occupational asthma, but in other contexts, as well the quantitative accuracy provided by the PEF meter, it may be able to expose triggers which are otherwise unnoticed.

OCCUPATIONAL ASTHMA

A patient's place of employment may (a) have caused the onset of asthma and/or (b) contain asthma triggers which exacerbate asthma. Both cases can be described as occupational asthma. When identified, cases of occupational asthma should be referred to a consultant. The reason for this referral is partly because of the effect of occupational asthma on a person's livelihood, but also because there may be inadequate care provided at the patient's place of work, and the patient may be in a position to obtain compensation. Initial identification of asthma is therefore important. Occupational asthma is detected in two ways: the effect of the work environment on PEF, and the effect of withdrawal from the work environment on PEF. In both cases, this involves careful monitoring of PEF, often at several times during the course of a day.

PEF varies throughout the day. As described in Chapter 1, PEF is lowest at night in the early hours of the morning and increases during the morning after waking, with a maximum sometime in the late afternoon. The effect of asthma triggers at work superimposes itself on this daily variation. Three patterns of occupational asthma can be identified: (a) the immediate reaction, (b) the late reaction and (c) the 'flat' record.

In the immediate reaction, the patient's PEF starts falling immediately on entering the work environment and starts to increase slightly on going home. Note how this is different from the normal daily pattern where PEF increases in the morning. In addition, in the case of the immediate reaction, the patient's PEF at home has a different daily pattern – i.e., does not show the decrease during the morning after waking. The immediate reaction is the kind of reaction described in the previous section as context specific PEF, and can easily be detected if the patient is able to measure PEF throughout the day on a couple of working week days and at a weekend.

In the late reaction, the drop in PEF starts at least an hour after entering the work place but may start several hours afterwards. For example, such a patient may show a fall in PEF starting in the early afternoon, and this fall continues into the evening, with a rise of PEF at night. Again the PEF record at the weekend is very different from that at work, and can be detected by regular daily readings (e.g., every 2 h).

The final pattern, the 'flat' record is the most difficult to detect, because there is no variation in PEF with work attendance and because there is actually very little PEF variation. Such a patient's PEF record appears similar to that in an irreversible lung disease such as chronic obstructive pulmonary disease. However, if the patient is removed from the work environment for more than 7 days, a gradual improvement in PEF occurs. This form of detection depends crucially on the patient's having a holiday, so holidays are important times if the patient is suspected of having occupational asthma. If occupational asthma is suspected, it is useful to plan some testing around the period of a holiday. Ideally the patient should take a PEF meter on holiday (and measure morning PEF throughout the holiday), but, as this may be difficult, the alternative is some careful testing on return and before the patient starts work again.

The immediate reaction, the delayed reaction and the 'flat' record describe types of occupational asthma which vary in severity or length of exposure, with the last being the most severe. Many kinds of workers are at risk from occupational asthma, which may account for 5% of adult-onset asthma, though some work environments may cause up to 50% of workers to be asthmatic. The list of people at risk is very wide but includes people working in the chemical industry (paints, adhesives, printing, photography, insulation products, metals), farmers and market gardeners (grain dust, pollens), millers and bakers (flour dust), paint sprayers, hair dressers and drug manufacturers.

PSYCHOLOGICAL FACTORS AND PEF

Psychological factors can affect the values obtained when using the PEF meter in four different ways: (a) measurement effects, (b) mood effects, (c) expectations and (d) relaxation effects. PEF measures the obstruction in the upper airways, so the relationship between psychological factors and PEF is limited to the upper airways.

Measurement effects

PEF is measured by patients blowing as hard as they can into a PEF meter. The value which is obtained by this procedure is effort dependent – which is why three blows are normally taken and the patient records the highest value. The effort put into the three blows may differ slightly. Evidently, if the patient does not feel like blowing hard, *all* those three values are going to be slightly less. Measurements of the relationship between psychological states and PEF are therefore subject to measurement error.

Patients who are tired or feel unwell may not blow as hard as the maximal possible. If there is variation in the effort expended, then this will lead to variation in PEF readings. A clinic assessment of PEF which produces substantially different values in the three blows should be approached with caution. It may be that the patient is not using maximal effort

In addition, patients are able to intentionally reduce the value of PEF by blowing less hard, though this is less common. However, if there is substantial variation in the three readings taken, then this may be the result of differences in level of effort – which may be caused by intentional under blowing.

In summary, although the PEF reading is often treated as some kind of gold standard, the health professional should be aware that the quality of the reading obtained depends crucially on motivational factors.

Mood effects

That negative mood acts as an asthma trigger has been discussed in earlier chapters. Unhappy moods, in particular those involving social conflicts, are particularly prone to cause bronchoconstriction. This effect is thought to be mediated via the vagal nerve, though other mediating pathways are possible – the underlying mechanism is not fully understood. Not all patients report that psychological factors act as a trigger; estimates vary depending on the criterion used, but at least one half show some sensitivity to mood states. Patients are particularly at risk from an asthma attack after a personal row or some other kind of emotionally stressful event. Of course if it were possible to predict rows, then it would be possible to increase preventative medicine in advance! However, the reality is that rows, like most other stresses, are normally unplanned, and therefore preventative action is not possible. Anecdotal evidence suggests that it is often *after* the stressful event has occurred that the patient notices deterioration of lung function. Whether this is a matter of recognition – people are too busy when rowing to notice symptoms – is unknown. Patients are not usually willing to measure their PEF for research purposes at regular intervals during a row.

The cause-and-effect relationship between mood and PEF works in both directions Poor lung function also has a negative effect on mood. Patients with poor PEF values often feel generally unwell, and their feelings can lead to suboptimal coping strategies. Some people, in particular those high in neuroticism, are likely to respond particularly badly to the emotional burden caused by poor PEF. Restoration of good lung function through initial aggressive treatment has the additional advantage of improving the patient's psychological wellbeing quickly. A quick improvement in mood is more likely to leave the patient feeling confident with the treatment – possibly leading to better coping strategies and compliance in the long term. Hence the recommended practice for dealing with a patient who is adversely affected by poor PEF is an initial aggressive treatment, followed by stepwise reduction.

Expectation effects

Some patients show measurable bronchodilation when they use a placebo bronchodilator. Some patients who are allergic to cats show measurable bronchoconstriction when they see a picture of a cat. Both examples illustrate the power of expectations: people's bodies tend to behave in the way they expect them to behave, where the expectations are based on past experience. The size of PEF changes caused by expectations varies between patients but can be up to 50% of the effect of an active pharmacological agent (see Sodergren & Hyland, in press, for a review).

Expectancy effects have not as yet proved to have any therapeutic value – regular use of placebo bronchodilators is not recommended! Nevertheless, the fact that expectancy effects occur may need to be taken into account, particularly when examining the effect of triggers on PEF: the trigger may not have to be physically present to have a triggering effect.

Relaxation effects

Because negative mood can have a bronchoconstricting effect, strategies to help patients cope with negative mood in stressful situations can be therapeutic in some cases. The research evidence (Vaquez & Buceta 1993) suggests that relaxation therapy can have a small but nevertheless significant beneficial effect in a certain proportion of patients. Benefits occur only in patients for whom psychological triggers play an important role, and the benefits include improved PEF and reduced reliever medication use. Relaxation therapy entails a sequence of training visits where the patient is taught how to relax and how to practise relaxation at home. After training, the patient can use this learned coping strategy when stressful events occur. The successful outcome of training is that stress has a smaller bronchoconstricting effect than previously. Relaxation training is therefore only suitable for patients where stress is recognised as being an important trigger.

PHYSICAL TRAINING

Although relaxation in asthma has been studied in the context of psychology, it also forms part of the physical training which may be provided as part of physiotherapy. It is interesting to note that, whereas in the UK asthma is managed primarily by doctors and nurses, in Scandinavian countries it tends to be managed by doctors and physiotherapists. Consequently, in those countries there tends to be a greater emphasis on physical training for asthma, which includes relaxation training for asthma attacks. In addition, physiotherapy aims to teach the patient good breathing habits, and to avoid the barrel chest that can arise from hyperinflation of the lungs.

Good general physical fitness is an advantage in asthma, but there are anecdotal reports and a very limited amount of research evidence that lung exercises can help. For example, it may be that taking up a wind instrument can help. The activity which appears to benefit the patient is the controlled breathing out of air, where expiration is under some resistance but inspiration is unimpeded (Singh 1987).

Box 5.9 Relaxation training for asthma attacks

The aim is to teach the patient how to experience relaxation and to use that experience to enable relaxation on the onset of an asthma attack. The patient is taught to focus on different parts of the body, relaxing each in turn. The patient is taught how to use diaphragmatic breathing and to find a position in which diaphragmatic breathing is comfortable (avoid lying on the back) such as sitting slumped forward or lying propped up on the side. The patient is taught that large volume breathing is tiring and so small volume or tidal breathing should be used. If the patient becomes familiar with these procedures, then they become easier to use in an asthma attack. Note that an asthma attack is arousing, and therefore it is easier to generate highly learned responses. Thus, there is merit in ensuring that the relaxation procedure is experienced regularly.

REFERRAL

The same asthma drugs can be prescribed by the general practitioner as are available through a respiratory consultant. Referral to a respiratory consultant is not done to achieve more powerful drugs – though patients may misunderstand this to be the case – but for other reasons having to do with patient management. There are five different reasons for referring a patient: diagnostic doubt, occupational asthma, management problems, severity, and limitation of expertise.

Diagnostic doubt

Asthma is not the only disease of the lungs. If there is any doubt about diagnosis then the patient should be referred to a respiratory consultant. The respiratory consultant will have a greater range of diagnostic equipment available and will be more experienced with less common lung diseases. Of course, doubt is something which varies in degree, but a safety-oriented policy would be to refer if doubt about the diagnosis crosses one's mind.

The BTS guidelines alert the health professional to the following areas of diagnostic doubt. First, patients who are elderly or who are smokers who have wheeze, and where there is the possibility of some other lung disease, such as chronic obstructive pulmonary disease. Second, those with unexplained persistent cough which may have a variety of causes, and finally patients with any systemic symptoms, such as fever, rash, weight loss, or proteinuria.

Occupational asthma

Occupational asthma has been described above, where it was noted that referral was needed not least because of legal implications for the patient and the employer. A respiratory or occupational consultant will be in a better position to advise and represent the patient's interests.

Management problems

If, despite the best endeavours of the primary care health professional, the patient still presents with problems or if the patients is responding poorly to advice (i.e., there are issues of noncompliance) then the patient should be referred. The BTS guidelines identify the following types of management problems:

1. those with sudden and catastrophic drops in PEF – called brittle asthma (note: those with brittle asthma are often provided by the specialist with an injector pen for emergencies)
2. those for whom increased therapy fails to reduce symptoms
3. those being considered for treatment with nebulised bronchodilators
4. pregnant women with worsening symptoms
5. patients who are experiencing unresolved quality-of-life problems
6. patients who have recently been discharged from hospital.

In summary, patients should be referred if inadequate control is being achieved, either in terms of quality of life or in terms of risk as indicated by emergency treatment. Patients who require frequent emergency care from the primary-care team, even if hospital attendance is not needed, should also be referred.

In referring patients on for these reasons the primary care health professional should not feel that he or she has failed in some way. Some patients simply want to see a consultant because they perceive that the consultant knows more and will therefore provide better care. Whether this is true or not is immaterial; the fact is that some patients actually want to be treated by a consultant, because going to the consultant is 'powerful medicine'. In addition, convergence of opinion between the consultant and primary-care professional may tip the balance for the patient towards better asthma management.

Severity

The North of England guidelines suggest that patients who are more severe should be referred, and certainly this makes sense for patients at Step 5 of the guidelines. Prescription of regular oral steroids is an important step in terms of side effect profile, and confirmation that it is necessary should be agreed with a specialist before embarking on this course of action. The North of England Guidelines also suggest that patients at Steps 3 and 4 should be referred. Although this would seem appropriate in many cases at Step 4, whether it becomes necessary at Step 3 should be discussed with the consultant as a matter of policy. Consultants become aware of differing levels of expertise in primary-care teams in their area and will therefore be able to offer appropriate advice to the particular practice.

Limitation of expertise

People don't become experts overnight. The ability to detect patterns in the patient's behaviour at an almost unconscious level – one of the characteristics of the expert – and the ability to respond to those patterns effectively, is something which develops over a period of time. Many forms of expertise cannot be learned from books! The primary-care health professional who is new to asthma management should not expect to have the skills of an experienced consultant, and it is important to be aware of the limitations of those skills. Patients should be referred if the health professional, experienced or otherwise, has doubt about the level of skill available in the primary-care setting to care for the patient, for whatever reason.

Asthma liaison nurse service

An asthma liaison nurse service is available in some areas of the country. The service provides liaison between secondary and primary care but is provided only for those patients admitted as inpatients or (in some cases) who attend an accident and emergency service for asthma. The asthma liaison service is staffed by experienced respiratory nurses working in association with respiratory consultants. The service is particularly helpful for patients with problems of compliance who may not attend the asthma clinic when requested.

CONCLUSIONS

This chapter has expanded on the idea of a self-management plan as introduced in the previous chapter. The main conclusion is that self-management plans need to be under constant review because of physiological and psychological changes that happen to the patient. Patients may need more or less anti-inflammatory medicine, and so the step of medication may need to be changed. In addition, there may be ways of optimising the amount of anti-inflammatory medicine needed, so that there can be refinements in the way action points are defined. Finally, there are issues relating to occupational asthma and psychological factors which may need to be considered for particular patients. However, in considering the various options, the health professional should not lose sight of something described in the last chapter. Some patients want to be empowered, to feel in control and to manage their own asthma. But some patients do not. The individualisation of management plans needs to be considered in relation to the patient's own preference for involvement.

REFERENCES

Beasley R, Cushley M, Holgate S T 1989 A self management plan in the treatment of adult asthma. Thorax 44: 200–204

British Asthma Guidelines Coordinating Committee 1997 British guidelines on asthma management: 1995 review and position statement. Thorax 52 (suppl.): S1–24

The British Thoracic Society and others 1993 Guidelines for the management of asthma. Thorax 48 (suppl.): S1–24

Charlton I, Charlton G, Broomfield J, Mullee M A 1990 Evaluation of peak flow and symptoms only self management plans for control of asthma in general practice. British Medical Journal 301: 1355–1359

Clark N M, Evans D, Mellins R E B 1992 Patient use of peak flow monitoring. American Review of Respiratory Disease 145: 722–725

Creer T L (in press) Home monitoring of lung function measures. In: Kotses H, Harver A (eds) Self-management of asthma. Marcel Dekker, New York

Gibson P G, Murree-Allen K, & Saltos N 1995 Annals of Internal Medicine 123: 488–492

Hyland M E, & Crocker G R 1995 Validation of an asthma quality of life diary in a clinical trial. Thorax 50: 724–730

International Consensus Report on Diagnosis and Treatment of Asthma 1992 National Institutes of Health (Publication No. 92–3091.), Bethesda, MD, USA.

Jones K P, Mullee M A, Middleton M, Chapman E, Holgate S T 1995 Peak flow based asthma self-management: a randomised controled study in general practice. Thorax 50: 851–857

Kendrick A M, Higgs C M B, Whitfield N J, Laszlo G 1993 Accuracy of perception of severity of asthma: patients treated in general practice. British Medical Journal 307: 422–424

Kikuchi Y, Okabe S, Tamura G, Hida W, Homma M, Shirato K, Takishima T 1994 Chemosensitivity and perception of dyspnea in patients with a history of near-fatal asthma. The New England Journal of Medicine 330: 1329–1334

McGee H M, O'Boyle C A, Hickely A, O'Malley K, Joyce C R B 1991 Assessing the quality of life of the individual: the SEOQoL with a health and a gastroenterology unit population. Psychological Medicine 21: 749–759

North of England Asthma Guideline Development Group 1996 North of England evidence based guidelines development project: summary version of evidence based guideline for the primary care management of asthma in adults. British Medical Journal 312: 762–766

Singh V 1987 Effect of respiratory exercises on asthma: the pink city lung exerciser. Journal of Asthma 24: 355–359

Sodergren, S C, Hyland M E (in press) Expectancy and asthma. In: Kirsch I (ed) Expectancy, experience, and behavior. APA Books, Washington, DC

Vaquez M I, Buceta J M 1993 Effectiveness of self-management programmes and relaxation training in the treatment of bronchial asthma: relationships with trait anxiety and emotional attack triggers. Journal of Psychosomatic Research 37: 71–81

Noncompliance and other problems

6

CONTENTS

WHAT IS 'NONCOMPLIANCE'?

Terminology

'Noncompliance' is really a rather unfortunate word. First, 'compliant' implies a rather passive, ineffectual sort of person, the sort of person who obeys without questioning. I am sure the average health professional would not want to be labelled 'compliant'. For this reason, some people object to the word 'compliance', and so alternative words such as 'adherence', 'cooperation' and 'concordance' are used instead. In this chapter I use the word compliance because, when I give health professionals the option during presentations, the majority tend to prefer that term. I personally do not have a preference either way. After a while 'adherence', 'cooperation' and 'concordance' end up meaning the same thing. Think how the word 'lavatory' (in Latin a place to wash) changes to 'toilet' (in French meaning a place to wash), and then changes into 'loo' and 'bathroom'. The human functions performed in these locations remains exactly the same despite the name changes.

The second reason why noncompliance is an unfortunate word is that the same word is used for very different things, and using the same word for different things can be confusing. The word 'noncompliance' is used if patients forget to take their inhaler, don't have the skill to use their MDI, or intentionally take less of their anti-inflammatory medicine than instructed. The word 'noncompliance' is used irrespective of whether the consequence of any of these actions puts the patient at risk or leads to a deterioration of quality of life. 'Noncompliance' is, in fact, a catch-all expression for a variety of different things – rather in the same way that 'quality of life' is a catch-all expression. This chapter has 'Noncompliance' in the title, but it is important to recognise the variety of behaviours, reasons and consequences that are associated with patients' not following their self management plans.

Box 6.1 Proportions of patients under- and overusing inhalers

Measurement of noncompliance has been greatly assisted by the development of electronic inhalers which have a chip inserted which records the time and date of use. Electronic records give different results to those from questionnaires – patients are seldom aware of overuse. In a study by Chemlik and Doughty (1994), patients on regular prophylactic medicine were given inhalers which had a small electronic chip placed inside. Chemlik and Doughty defined compliance as 'being within 10% of the recommended dose'. After patients had used the inhalers for a time, the researchers found that the percentage of compliant and noncompliant patients was:

- compliant 40%
- underusers 50%
- overusers 10%.

The behaviours of noncompliance

A number of research studies show that, of patients on regular prophylactic medicine, about half take less than the recommended dose and a small number take more than recommended (Box 6.1). Noncompliance, far from being an infrequent occurrence, is something that occurs in at least 50% of asthma patients. This is a sobering thought. Patients often do not self-manage as recommended.

The distinction of underusers versus overusers does not, however, capture the full range of noncompliant behaviours. Some patients have a cyclical pattern of underuse and overuse. Others have an erratic pattern with occasional underuse, or underuse on particular occasions (for example, 'drug holidays' at the weekend).

Another important behavioural pattern of noncompliance is where the patient fails to respond to action points in an appropriate way. A patient may take the correct amount of prophylactic medicine regularly but not increase the dose when symptoms deteriorate. Equally, the patient may delay visiting the clinic or hospital when symptoms are sufficiently bad for the patient to seek help. Thus, noncompliance is not simply a matter of underuse of steroids. Noncompliance (or nonadherence, or noncooperation or nonconcordance) is a shorthand expression for any form of patient self-management inconsistent with the advice being given by the health professional.

Reasons for non-compliance

It is usual to divide the *reasons* for noncompliance into two categories (Royal Pharmaceutical Society 1996):

1. unintentional noncompliance where the patient unintentionally self-manages in a way other than recommended
2. intentional noncompliance where the patient intentionally self-manages in a way other than recommended.

Although this distinction is a useful starting point, the difference between intended and nonintended noncompliance is less clear than appears at first sight. Intention implies that the patient is doing something consciously, and there are certainly instances where this is the case in noncompliance. Equally, nonintentional implies that the patient is not consciously failing to comply. However, as we shall see later in the chapter, there are instances where the patient's insight into behaviour is uncertain and the distinction between intentional and nonintentional noncompliance is less useful.

Consequences of noncompliance

Noncompliance is associated with greater asthma morbidity (Horn, Clark & Cochrane 1990), and is therefore undesirable for physiological reasons. Of course, this does not mean that all noncompliance is associated with greater asthma morbidity, but the association does indicate that at least some noncompliance creates physiological problems. In particular, acute admissions and asthma death often involve poor management in the form of noncompliance, and so the topic should be treated seriously by health professionals.

It has been said that noncompliance is a hidden epidemic in health care, because it happens in almost all medical contexts, and particularly those involving prevention. In fact, noncompliance in asthma is no more frequent than in many other diseases, and the consequences can be less severe. In the case of successful organ transplants, the majority of subsequent rejections occur because patients do not take their immunosuppressant drugs – though patients seldom admit it to the doctor when requesting a new transplant. There is no going back once organ rejection sets in following even a short period of noncompliance. Noncompliance in asthma is frequently less dramatic – though it can be fatal.

Can noncompliance be predicted?

It is extremely difficult to predict which patients are compliant or not. Bender and Milgrom (1996) found that only 50% of predictions of compliance by a physician were correct. Some asthma record cards have a category for 'compliance', which is indicated as either 'good' or 'poor'. Such records have minimal use. Not only is the term 'compliance' too general, but the health professional will be inaccurate in many cases. There are certain 'at risk' groups who are more likely to fail to comply than others, and these will be described later in the chapter. However, it is important not to use a simple stereotype in deciding who is noncompliant. Some people from low-risk groups fail to comply, whereas others from high-risk groups follow their self-management plan thoroughly.

In trying to predict noncompliance in asthma, it is useful to consider other treatments. Interestingly, one drug where compliance is extremely good is the contraceptive pill, and the reason for this is something we should bear in mind when examining asthma compliance. Clearly, compliance depends crucially on the patient's understanding of the purpose for which the therapy is being taken, and the consequences of not taking it. The example of the contraceptive pill shows that good compliance is possible.

In summary, when trying to understand noncompliance, three related sets of questions need to be addressed:

1. What exactly does the noncompliant behaviour amount to?
2. What are the reasons for the behaviour? Why is it actually occurring?
3. What is the consequence of noncompliance? Does it impact on the patient's quality of life? Does it make the patient less safe? Does it make any difference?

Each of these questions will be considered in the following sections.

FORGETTING, MISUNDERSTANDING AND TECHNIQUE

The best way to deal with the kind of noncompliance described in this section is to focus on the way the self-management plan has been devised and communicated – blaming the patient may be accurate but doesn't help matters!

Forgetting to take the medicine

In Chapter 4, I suggested that, as part of their self-management plan, patients should be told what to do if they forget to take their medicine. Some degree of forgetting is to be expected, but patients are more likely to forget to take their medicine if they are high in neuroticism (Ch. 3) or if their cognitive ability is poor (Ch. 3). Quite simply, there is what could be called an 'incompetence factor', and some patients are not very competent at managing the medicine. Rather than just forgetting to take the medicine, some patients may forget that they have taken it and so take more doses than recommended.

There are several possible strategies open to the health professional if forgetting to take the medicine is so frequent that it becomes a health problem. One way is to increase the feedback to the patient. Feedback provides information about whether forgetting has occurred. For example, in the case of the contraceptive pill, where compliance is in fact excellent, the days are labelled so that patients know whether they have taken the dose on a particular day. This form of labelling is not common with current asthma devices, but the health professional may find that prescribing a device which provides good feedback to the patient is helpful if forgetting is common (either failing to take enough or taking too many doses).

A second strategy is to provide advice about lifestyle which may increase the likelihood of remembering. For example, the patient should be advised how to use regular everyday occurrences (such as teeth brushing) as a reminder, though the particular everyday occurrences involved will need to be discussed with the patient.

The consequences of forgetting depend on the amount of missed doses as well as on the physiological characteristics of the patient. For patients with severe asthma and whose asthma is only just adequately controlled by the prescribed medication, the effects are likely to be more severe. However, for many other patients, the effect of forgetting may be less severe in that inhaled steroids are reasonably 'forgiving' of forgetting (Ch. 4). However, care needs to be taken in communicating this point to the patient, to prevent 'unintentional' forgetting merging imperceptibly into 'intentional' forgetting.

Because the effects of forgetting vary considerably between patients, the significance of forgetting can be assessed in terms of exacerbations. If patients require regular rescue treatment (courses of oral steroids, out-of-hours visits, hospital attendance), it is worth exploring whether recent forgetting of inhaled steroids has contributed.

Forgetting the instructions

As discussed in Chapter 4, the health professional should, as part of routine management, help patients memorise instructions (e.g., provide written instruction leaflets). Nevertheless, there is a minority of patients for whom instructions are easily forgotten because of the cognitive ability of the patient. Forgetting takes a variety of forms. It may be a confusion between the action of the 'blue' and 'brown' inhaler. It may be forgetting when to increase steroid dose, or when to seek assistance. It may be forgetting to come to the asthma clinic.

For such 'forgetful' patients it is important to make the self-management plan as simple as possible. When simplifying the self-management plan, some degree of patient empowerment is traded off against ease of comprehension, but that may not pose a problem for the less cognitively able patient. Simple plans with a comfortable margin of error in the level of regular steroid prescribed may work more effectively.

The consequences of forgetting the instructions again depend on the physiology of the patient. For example, a patient who uses the blue inhaler twice a day and the brown one when symptomatic may indeed end up with a dose of anti-inflammatory medicine only slightly less than that prescribed, though too much bronchodilator. Such a patient would, of course, have a pattern of anti-inflammatory medication that lags behind the development of inflammation, so this pattern of medication is not optimal. The patient who forgets whom to contact and what to do in an emergency, however, is considerably more at risk.

Inappropriate instructions

Patients can interpret what is said to them literally, rather than applying what the health professional considers to be common sense. Earlier, I gave the example of a patient who would miss out on her evening prophylactic medicine if she went to bed before 6 o'clock, because she had been told to take it after 6 p.m. There are many other accounts of patient misunderstandings which illustrate the innovative ways in which patients can misinterpret instructions. For example, consider the case of a newly diagnosed patient who was told by her doctor that she ought to get rid of her cat if she could, but in any case he would give her an asthma inhaler to use twice per day. The woman would spray the inhaler on the cat, morning and evening, as she thought she had been instructed, because she didn't want to get rid of her cat. Or take the case of a couple where the elderly, pipe-smoking husband was diagnosed as having asthma. The doctor suggested to the wife that it would help if the husband stopped smoking, and prescribed an asthma inhaler to be used morning and evening. The husband would sit grumpily in his chair smoking in the morning and evening, while the wife hovered around and gave him a couple of squirts with the inhaler.

If you think this kind of problem cannot happen to you, think again. Patients may be given the right instructions, but the occasional patient will still end up doing something other than that intended. Careful assessment of the patient's lifestyle (Ch. 3), and subsequent checking of behaviour, may help detect this problem where it occurs. In this, as with other reasons for noncompliance discussed in this section, the remedy depends on the health professional's being able to detect that there is a problem. Patients seldom detect their own misinterpretations!

Box 6.2 Example of misinterpretation of instructions

A very experienced respiratory nurse (who is also a trainer for the National Asthma and Respiratory Training Centre) told me the following story. She told a patient to take oral steroids if her PEF ever reached 200. Some time afterwards, the patient was admitted to hospital with a much lower PEF. When the patient was asked why she hadn't taken any steroids, the patient said 'Well it never actually got to 200. It was 220, and then it went down to 180 and then it went down a bit more, but it was never 200' . No comment is needed!

Technique

Poor technique can lead to inadequate amounts of drug being inhaled. As a general rule, the more recent devices have been designed to avoid some of the problems of poor technique, but not all problems can be avoided by design. The following problems are associated with the 'standard' (i.e., older style) MDI, and devices which overcome the problem are also described.

1. *Failure to coordinate actuation with breathing in* This problem is surprisingly common, one researcher reporting that about 50–60% of people naive to an MDI have a problem in coordination (Crompton 1988). The problem of coordination is dealt with by breath-actuated MDIs, dry powder inhalers, and standard inhalers with a spacer. Visual inspection by the health professional will indicate whether it is occurring or not, but testing devices are also available.

2. *The 'cold freon' effect* in which the patient closes the back of the

mouth and breathes in through the nose when the cold gas from the inhaler strikes the inside of the mouth. This problem is much more difficult to detect, because the patient still appears to be breathing in. Electronic testing devices can show whether inhalation through the mouth continues. Some patients find it very difficult not to respond with a cold freon effect even when they understand what the problem is. Devices designed to overcome the cold freon effect include a vortex MDI which produces gas at a slower exit speed, dry powder inhalers, and standard MDIs with spacer.

3. *Failure to expire properly prior to inhalation.* This problem is easy to detect with visual inspection, but no device is designed to overcome it. Repeated advice to the patient may be necessary.

4. *Failure to hold breath after inspiration.* Again, the problem is easy to detect, no device is designed to overcome it, and repeated advice may be necessary.

Research on the adequacy of inhaler technique makes for dismal reading, and leads to the conclusion that the first thing to check if a patient is not well controlled is whether adequate amounts of drug are actually getting into the lungs. The standard MDIs have the poorest record for technique, and dry powder inhalers and the more recent MDIs were designed largely to overcome the deficiency of the standard MDI. However, even dry powder inhalers have their problems. One study examining technique with a dry powder inhaler came to the conclusion that only 5% of patients had good technique, 78% were adequate, and 27% were insufficient (Dompeling et al 1992). In their investigation of patients 4 months after intensive instruction, only 3 out of 41 patients expired adequately prior to inspiration, and 22 of the 41 did not make any attempt to hold breath after inspiration.

These data indicate that poor technique may be more common than expected, and that regular checking of technique is needed.

CONSCIOUS DECISIONS NOT TO FOLLOW INSTRUCTIONS

Overview of intentional noncompliance

Providing the patient with information which is correctly understood does not always lead to compliance (Blessing-Moore 1996). A correct understanding of asthma is a necessary condition to achieve compliance, and it is certainly worthwhile – but it is not sufficient.

Intentional noncompliance occurs when the patient makes a decision not to follow the self-management plan recommended by the health professional. This decision may be taken in the asthma clinic while the recommendation is being made, or the decision may be made at some later stage when the patient decides, after all, not to follow the instructions. In coming to this decision, the patient may either be well informed or be poorly informed and make a judgement on incorrect information. Whatever the physiological outcome of intentional noncompliance – not all intentional noncompliance is dangerous – the psychological consequence is negative. If the patient is unable to tell the health professional that instructions are not being followed, if the patient is unable to negotiate an acceptable self-management plan with the health professional, then this detracts from the relationship between the health professional and patient. Intentional noncompliance means conscious deception. People find it difficult to trust those whom they have deceived, just as those we dislike most are often those to whom we have done the greatest harm. So intentional noncompliance will lead to the patient's failing to trust the health professional – and not just the other way round.

Cost–benefit analysis is an approach to decision making where a person weighs up the advantages and disadvantages of a particular course of action, and only carries out that action if the advantages outweigh the disadvantages. People, and not just patients, weigh up the costs and benefits of actions and come to a rational decision on the basis of all the evidence, including what other people are doing.

There are several different theories of cost–benefit analysis theory which have been applied to health care. The best known of these is

Box 6.3 Bear this in mind!

I have on my wall something said to me by an asthmatic student, several years ago. This is what she said about the way she managed her asthma:

'I don't go by what doctors tell me. I have seen so many, and they all told me different things. I just go by what is right for me. Also, they only understand asthma from books. They don't really know what it is like.'

the Health Beliefs Model (Rosenstock 1974). According to this model, healthy behaviour is promoted or inhibited by:

1. the perceived likelihood of a negative outcome occurring
2. the severity of the negative event
3. the benefits of preventative actions
4. barriers to performing preventative action.

Thus, according to this and similar models, the patient's decisions about asthma management depend on a rational answer to the question, 'What are the advantages and what are the disadvantages of following the self-management instructions?'. There are a large number of advantages and disadvantages of asthma compliance which are listed in this section and will be discussed under two categories: practical considerations and health beliefs.

Practical considerations

Inconvenience

It is inconvenient to take medicine on a regular basis. If a person is very busy, then taking medicine is a nuisance, and the nuisance is compounded if the patient is also asked to measure PEF. Drugs which are taken four times a day (e.g., sodium cromoglycate) are less convenient than drugs which are taken twice a day (e.g., beclomethasone), and patients 'comply' less well with the four times a day regimen than the twice a day. Whether this is due to forgetting or to intentional undermedication is unclear, but clearly, a four times a day regimen is less convenient. A once a day inhaler is more convenient than the twice a day inhaler, though there is no clear

Box 6.4 Compliance and frequency of dosing

There is surprisingly little research on the advantage of different frequencies of dosing. However, one study of compliance with anti-epileptic drugs reported 87% compliance with once per day, 81% compliance with twice per day, 77% compliance with three times per day, and 39% compliance with four times per day (Cramer et al 1989). This study is often quoted to support the contention that twice a day is better than four times a day, but there is not much difference between once a day and twice a day. In fact the sample sizes were small, and the results may not be very informative for clinical practice.

evidence showing this to have an advantage in terms of the total amount of compliance. On the other hand, a once a day routine may be preferred by some patients.

Budesonide has been licensed for once a day use, where double the morning or evening dose is taken only on one occasion during the day. In fact, there is no reason why beclomethasone or fluticasone could not be used in the same way. The evidence with budesonide is that there is no significant difference between the twice a day and once a day routine in moderate patients in terms of standard outcome measures. Other research shows that taking steroids more regularly throughout the day leads to a greater anti-inflammatory effect. However, if the level of steroid at a less frequent dose regimen provides comfortably adequate protection then there may be no advantage in having the more frequent dose regimen. It would seem sensible, therefore, to consider the once a day regimen only for patients with moderate asthma (e.g., Step 2).

In deciding whether to recommend a once a day regimen, the health professional needs to consider two factors. First, is the patient inconvenienced by the twice a day regimen? Does the patient actually prefer it or will it make no difference? There needs to be a clear advantage to the patient for the once a day regimen to be recommended. Second, how often does the patient forget? The consequence of forgetting on any one occasion on a twice a day regimen is less than the consequence of forgetting on one occasion on a once a day regimen. Patients who regularly forget to take their inhaler – unless they do so only in the evening or morning – should not be recommended the once daily routine. Although the manufacturers of budesonide recommend that patients should take their inhaler once daily in the evening, there is in fact no evidence to support once a day evening versus once a day morning use. In sum, the use of inhalers once a day should be considered if inconvenience is a problem to patients.

The design of the inhaler device is another factor which affects convenience. Some dry powder inhalers are very fiddly to use. Large spacers can be inconvenient to carry around. The convenience of different devices should be discussed with the patient. There is no point in prescribing a device which the patient is not going to use. In discussing this point, one should note that the intention to comply in the clinic may be very real. The problem occurs after the clinic visit, when intentions can change. Thus, convenience of devices needs to be assessed on subsequent visits:

Nurse: 'How are you getting on with your inhaler?'

Patient 'It's okay.'

Nurse: 'Do you find it a bother to use?'

Patient: 'Well it's not too bad.'

Nurse: 'If you find it a real bother, we can work out something which may make it easier for you. We can look at it again next time if you like.'

Selecting a device for the patient is just as important as selecting the right drug. Not all patients get on well with the same device, and so preference may need to be explored. Allegiance to one manufacturer restricts patient choice!

Patients are unlikely to admit that inconvenience is the root cause of noncompliance without considerable encouragement. Patients do not like admitting that they can't be bothered to follow the health professional's instructions, because that implies that they do not value what the health professional has told them.

Side effects and risks

A second disadvantage of regular prophylactic medicine is the perceived or real side effects or risks associated with regular medicine taking. Perceived side effects and the perceived risks of an asthma attack versus overmedication will be discussed in a later section. However, it is worth noting that some patients do experience side effects, and the experience of those side effects will almost certainly impair compliance with treatment. In particular, if patients on high-dose inhaled steroids at Step 3 of the BTS guidelines are experiencing side effects, then there are several options available (see Ch. 5) and the health professional should consider those options. Every effort should be made to avoid side effects, as they will decrease the likelihood of compliance.

Financial costs

For patients who pay prescription charges, asthma medicine imposes a financial cost which depends on the number and frequency of medicines used. It is worth noting that diabetics do not pay for their medicines, whereas asthmatics do – a fact which appears anomalous, at least to those who are, or are involved with, asthmatics. Cost is a much greater burden on patients than is often appreciated. In one survey (Hyland et al 1995), cost was the second most important asthma bother for those patients who paid for their prescription.

Patients respond to the financial cost in several ways. One patient, a health professional, takes half the recommended dose as an economy measure. Others go to the pharmacist and say 'I can only afford one of these, which do you suggest?'. Some only submit the prescription for the bronchodilator medicine because 'that is the one that seems to work best'.

Detecting and managing noncompliance due to cost is particularly problematic because patients will take their prescriptions from the clinic, and consequently, in terms of the clinic record, the evidence suggests that the patient is taking their medicine. As with any form of intentional noncompliance, patients find it difficult to admit that they are not taking their medicine, but restriction based on cost is particularly difficult to admit to. On the one hand such an admission implies poverty or incompetence or both. On the other it implies placing less value on health care than on other activities, such as going to the cinema, and the patient feels that this undervaluation of health care will not square with the health professional's own values. It is like saying, I don't really think that what you tell me is important. The ability to detect and manage cost-related noncompliance depends on a good relationship between the health professional and patient. Questions such as:

> 'Do you find the cost of these medicines a real bother?'

can be a useful starting point, followed by

> 'I know some people actually don't take all their medicine because of cost.'

It may be best to leave it to the patient to respond or not as the case may be. A confrontational question such as 'Are you so poor and

Box 6.5

In a standard 250-actuation MDI the MDI will continue working after the 250 doses but the dose is actually very variable – and often less. Some patients require emergency treatment when they have 'run out' of their prophylactic medicine. It may be that they actually 'ran out' of adequate doses some time back, but thought that the prophylactic inhaler was providing adequate doses simply because it was working.

ignorant that you can't afford these wonderful medicines?' is unlikely to help, and although I am sure no one would ask that directly, it is important not to give the same impression by innuendo.

If cost does restrict use of inhalers, particularly the anti-inflammatory inhalers, then the health professional should explore ways of increasing the number of doses available to the patient per prescription paid.

Short-term versus long-term benefit

Patients are advised that prophylactic medicine has long-term benefits, whereas short-acting β-agonists have only short-term benefits. However, for many people, long benefits are discounted in the sense that they are not thought to be very important. Some people evaluate events primarily for the present, and will not plan for the future. Such patients will undervalue the advantages of prophylactic medicine in relation to their short-acting β-agonists, and the argument that anti-inflammatory medicine has long-acting benefits will be valued differently by the patient and the health professional.

The use of a combined medicine (i.e. a β-agonist combined with a steroid) may be useful for patients who undervalue and so fail to use their prophylactic medicine. Although I have heard of informal reports that a combined preparation (e.g., Ventide) improves outcome in some patients, the research evidence does not in fact support this (Bosley, Parry & Cochrane 1994), and, because of that evidence, combined preparations are not currently recommended.

Health beliefs

General health beliefs

Health beliefs are the beliefs a patient has about disease, medicines and how medicines work on the body. Patients have general health beliefs as well as disease-specific beliefs, i.e., in the present case, beliefs about asthma. A person's beliefs about asthma will be influenced to a large extent by their general beliefs.

Some people have a general belief that it is 'bad' to have medicine. If you ask a patient:

> 'If you have a headache would you take an aspirin or paracetamol, or would you prefer to manage without?'

the answer to this question will give a fairly good idea about the patient's general orientation to drug treatment. There are several reasons for an antipathy towards taking drugs of any description. For some people, taking a medicine is a sign of weakness. Others respond in a way which emphasises the idea of 'naturalness': it just isn't natural to take drugs. It is natural for the body to heal itself. For others it is the unknown side effects, or the risk of the unknown, which is the motivation to avoid treatment. Fear of the unknown can be a powerful motivator for avoidance. Questions about the patient's attitude towards nonasthma drugs are often useful and revealing. The patient feels less threatened explaining why aspirin is avoided, rather than saying why asthma drugs are avoided, but the behaviour and reason are likely to be similar in both cases.

General beliefs about the body and treatment provide some information about asthma beliefs, but they are useful to know for another reason. Asthma beliefs are held in the context of these other beliefs, and it is for this contextual reason that asthma beliefs are resistant to change. To change asthma beliefs, it may be necessary to change the general beliefs as well – which is difficult – or, at least, to change the way asthma beliefs relate to general beliefs. For some patients, this may be difficult.

Steroid phobia

Steroid are a particular class of drugs which are used in asthma, and if patients do not like taking drugs, they will also prefer to avoid steroids. However, steroids are drugs for which there are specific beliefs which lead to their avoidance. As discussed previously, there is a degree of negative media coverage of steroids, and negative accounts of oral steroids (for example, when used by athletes) are confused with inhaled steroids.

When dealing with steroid phobic patients, one approach to take, particularly with standard-dose inhaled steroids, is to say that the medicine is perfectly safe. Whether or not it is safe is immaterial. The fact is that communicating in this way has low credibility. As a general rule, people do not believe arguments which are contrary to their own beliefs if they are presented in a one-sided manner. 'Double-barrelled' communications – where both sides of the argument are put – are much more effective in dealing with patients who hold views contrary to what is being advised.

How should one proceed with double-barrelled communication in steroid phobic patients? The are a number of strategies, but the following illustrates a possible approach.

> 'Obviously, taking steroids isn't good; even in the very minute amounts that are inhaled. The asthma guidelines recommend that you use as little as is necessary to control your inflammation.' (This is perfectly true – see the 1997 guidelines.) 'The amount which is prescribed is the minimum we can get away with. No one wants to prescribe any more drugs than are absolutely necessary. But any less, and then you are at risk for asthma attacks and damage caused by inflammation. I know it is not ideal, but taking it really is the better option for your health overall.'

Notice how this style of communication makes the patient's concern over steroids legitimate. Legitimising concerns is a first step in overcoming those concerns. Statements such as:

> 'Of course you are worried about it. It is perfectly natural to worry'

are surprisingly effective for communicating with worried patients, and not only patients who are worried about their asthma.

Beliefs about risk

There are two sorts of risk associated with asthma medicine: the risk of present or future side effects (i.e., the risk of overmedication), and the risk of insufficient control leading to an asthma attack or death (i.e., the risk of undermedication). Although there are objective risks associated with any one patient, the *perceived* risks may be very different, and it is the perceived risks that determine the patient's behaviour.

Box 6.6 Assessing patient's perceptions of risk

An indication of the patient's perceptions of risk can be found from answers to the following sorts of question:

- the risk of undermedication leading to exacerbations and possibly death:

  'How worried are you about having an asthma attack?'

- the risk of overmedication leading to present or future adverse health effects:

  'If you have a headache, do you take an aspirin or paracetemol, or do you prefer to try to manage without?' 'What do you feel about steroids?'

Some patients will be more concerned about the risk of undermedication and some about the risk of overmedication. The greater the perceived risk of undermedication, the more likely the patient is to take the prescribed medication. However, if the perceived risk of undermedication is high and the perceived risk of overmedication very low, then the patient may take more medicine than required. Recall from the example given at the beginning of the chapter that, although the majority of noncompliance involves undermedication, 10% of patients were taking too much prophylactic medicine. There are a small number of patients who, when told to double their steroid dose when symptomatic, double it all the time. The logic of doing so is that the double dose must be safe (or it wouldn't have been prescribed) so why risk having any inconvenience from asthma? Careful monitoring of steroid use will detect both over- and underuse.

The perceived risk of undermedication is influenced by the patient's perception of whether they have asthma. Some patients say:

> 'I don't really have asthma. I just sometimes have asthma attacks'.

This is an interesting statement because not only does it indicate denial of the diagnosis, but also that asthma is a disease which is located somewhere outside the person. It is a disease which happens to the patient, rather than something within the patient's control.

In fact, the perception that asthma is a disease outside the patient and which is responded to only when it 'hits' the patient is consistent with how patients perceive the cause and management of many other diseases. For example, when patients develop a sore throat, they can believe that the cause is external, i.e., they picked up some sore throat bacteria from outside, and so they go to the doctor and ask for a course of antibiotics to kill the bacteria. In the same way, going to the A & E department for asthma treatment reflects the belief that asthma is something which is visited upon people for no apparent reason from outside, just like sore throats.

When explaining asthma to patients, it can be useful to emphasise that asthma does not work like common complaints such as sore throats. However, one difficulty in convincing patients that asthma is not an occasional acute illness is that they will often feel perfectly well between asthma attacks. Hence, the feeling of wellness is inconsistent with the statement, provided by the health professional, that the patient's body is ill and needs treatment.

It can be difficult to convince patients about the need for regular treatment when they have strongly held beliefs about the externality of asthma, but one possible approach to dealing with this problem is to focus the patient's attention on the kind of relationship that occurs between PEF and symptomatology. If the relationship is poor, and symptoms are poor predictors of exacerbations, then this fact may be demonstrated to the patient to illustrate that the feeling of wellness does not show all is well. However, as noted in Chapter 3, the perception of illness as something which is outside the body is often based on a desire to preserve self-esteem, and as this motivation is one of the strongest, it may be very difficult to get denying patients to accept that they have asthma, other than in a superficial sense and to please the health professional. For a minority of cases, it may be necessary to accept the patient's unchanging perception of what asthma is and adopt a self management plan which enables the patient to manage the asthma, with frequent monitoring, on a more variable basis. In particular, for such patients, it may be necessary to have a more conservative action point for when assistance is needed. For example, the action point for A & E attendance may be increased from 50% to 60% of best – or whatever method of determining the action point is adopted (see Ch. 5).

Denial of asthma decreases the patient's perceived risk of undermedication, but information from the media and from family and friends may increase the perceived risk of overmedication. Throughout society, people vary in their perception of the risk of conventional drugs, and this perception forms part of a culture within which the patient lives. For some patients, their anxiety about

Box 6.7 The relationship between perceived risk and precautions

Patients are more likely to take their medicine if they perceive asthma to be a *serious* illness. But the perception of having a serious illness affects self-esteem and detracts from quality of life. An alternative perspective is to think of asthma as a non-serious but potentially dangerous condition, and a useful analogy of this perspective is that of a car. A car is potentially dangerous. If the brakes aren't checked and the tyres replaced when worn, then the car is just as dangerous as asthma, if not more so. But people do not worry, every time they drive their car, whether it is safe, even though they check their brakes and tyres regularly.

risk of overmedication is maintained by contact with other people, not necessarily having asthma, who have either positive or negative attitudes towards the potential risk of regular medicine. Within this context, it is worth noting that 'replacement' of what is natural is not seen as a risk – for example, people can quite happily overdose on vitamins. The perceived risk of overmedication is increased by perceptions that steroids are an unnatural addition, as opposed to a 'replacement' that maintains health. In addition, correct reports about inappropriate use of oral steroids appear in the press and give rise to a general negative feeling about steroids.

Cultural differences in beliefs about medicine and asthma treatment

People from ethnic minority groups have a higher than average rate of hospital admission for asthma despite having average prevalence (Ayres 1986, Omerod 1995), and it seems likely that management may be particularly problematic in these groups. Education targeted specifically to ethnic minorities has been found to be helpful in the USA (Fisher et al 1994). Awareness of cultural characteristics and background is therefore important when managing patients from a different cultural background to one's own.

As emphasised above, beliefs about asthma occur in the context of more general beliefs about disease, and this occurs as much in the white majority as in ethnic populations. However, ethnic populations often have systems of medicine and health beliefs which are well developed and respected in their own communities. Ethnic populations have their own, traditional medicines. It often happens that traditional medicines are practised side by side with western medicines (Bhopal 1986), and this is likely to be the case with asthma as with any other disease. For example, the patient may go to the GP on one day, and go to the acupuncturist on another – but not necessarily telling one about the other. Although this mix of two parallel treatments for asthma is not in itself bad, problems arise when the western asthma medicine is discontinued and the traditional medicine retained. For example, suppose an Asian patient starts taking regular western prophylactic medicine but also takes turmeric in milk as treatment for asthma. If the asthma symptoms disappear, their disappearance may be attributed to the turmeric, so it would be perfectly natural to discontinue the western medicine, which is more expensive! It is unrealistic to expect people from ethnic minority groups to easily reject their own medicine in favour of western medicine. The traditional medicine of the ethnic minority group is part of their culture, it is reinforced by other members of their (often) close-knit families, and is further reinforced by contact with friends and family from overseas.

Box 6.8 An analogy to the accommodation of traditional medicine

Both in past and more recent times, Christian missionaries have worked on the principle that it is better to incorporate native beliefs into Christianity rather than try to reject them outright. It is no accident that the European pagan winter solstice festival coincides with Christmas and that the pagan spring festival coincides with Easter. Similarly, Christian practice in Africa includes native rituals from indigenous religions. Health professionals can learn a useful lesson from missionaries – perhaps their work is not that different. It may be better to incorporate the traditional medicine into the asthma care of the patient, rather than to try to reject it outright.

Each minority group has its own set of beliefs, and there can be differences between people from apparently similar backgrounds. For example, different Asian groups have different health beliefs. The best approach to finding out about a patient's beliefs is to ask patients directly. Expressions of interest in other people's medical practice often meet with a positive response. The following is illustrative of the kind of ethnic beliefs that exist.

Chinese medicine is based on the principle of 'balance' between different types of life force, and treatment includes not only acupuncture and herbal remedies but also diet and lifestyle. A similar emphasis on the principle of balance is found in the Ayurvedic tradition of Asia (India and Pakistan) where, as in Chinese medicine, western medicine is perceived as very powerful in the short term but contributing to long-term imbalance. Hence there can be a conflict between taking the 'hot' steroids of western medicine and the balance which is sought through traditional means. Asian treatments include yoga and diet; diet may involve spices, including ginger, karela, and garlic. Afro-Caribbean medicines consist primarily of herbs, roots and 'bitters' sometimes obtained from the Caribbean.

The efficacy of these traditional medicines is difficult to evaluate. In fact, some Chinese herbs contain steroids – so the herbs may not be as innocuous as one might imagine.

In Chinese medicine, substances taken in through the lungs are 'bad' whereas substances taken in through the mouth are 'good'. People from Eastern cultures, in particular from Japan and China, may have difficulty seeing that inhalers are 'good'. It seems no accident that the first anti-leukotriene to be launched onto a medical market (a tablet anti-inflammatory medicine) was launched in Japan.

In addition to a different medical philosophy and practice, patients from ethnic minorities may prefer to interact with health professionals in a way which differs from that of the majority population. In some minority groups the preferred level of control may be different from that in the majority population. In some Asian groups, for example, there is a greater tendency for the patient to expect the health professional to 'sort out the asthma' rather than become actively involved in self-management. Hence, giving a high degree of empowerment to such a patient will result in a failure to follow the self-management plan. But this does not apply to all Asians – the lesson to be learned is that one needs to pay particular attention to assessing the patient's preferred level of control.

Box 6.9 Example of the influence of a cultural attitude

I once spoke to a Japanese consultant about compliance. 'We don't have noncompliance here' he said. 'Actually, we probably do, but noncompliance is looked on as such an insult to the physician, that to admit to it would involve terrible loss of face. We just can't investigate it.'

Finally, the meaning of asthma may be different in ethnic minority cultures. For example, the diagnosis of a chronic illness may be stigmatising and have implications for future marriage. Considerable sensitivity to the implications of having asthma is needed, particularly when communicating with relatives of the asthma patient.

In dealing with ethnic minority groups, it is important not to jump to premature conclusions on the basis of skin colour. Many people from ethnic minorities have integrated into the majority culture: ethnic minority status implies an additional obligation to assess, rather than a foregone conclusion about the patient's beliefs.

Complementary medicines and diet

Of course, a patient does not have to come from an ethnic minority to believe in and practice traditional medicine. Many patients from all backgrounds have a positive attitude towards complementary medicines of all kinds. Indeed, an inspection of the self-help books on asthma in a local bookshop will show how popular complementary approaches are.

Complementary medicines which may be used with asthma include homeopathy, acupuncture, yoga, Chinese herbal remedies, as well as dietary and lifestyle changes, but may extend to aromatherapy and foot massage. Are these treatments effective? The answer is that we don't really know, though the efficacy of some complementary treatments is likely to be less than others (aromatherapy, for example, would not feature high in a list of likely treatments). The reason for the lack of knowledge is that inadequate research has been done, though a large homeopathy study is currently underway in the Southampton area and the results will be available soon. Available research for acupuncture and yoga is reviewed in the North of England guidelines, but the authors conclude that there is no evidence to support the use of these treatments alone. The reason for the scarcity of research is complex, but has to do, at least in part, with the different conceptual approach taken by complementary practitioners and the researchers who represent the western tradition. For example, in both Chinese medicine (herbs and acupuncture) and homeopathy, a distinction is made between different types of asthma which have different causes and so should be treated differently. This belief makes it difficult to investigate efficacy using the conventional 'randomised clinical trial' where there is an implicit assumption of uniformity of disease between patients.

Nevertheless, there are anecdotal reports from some patients that complementary treatments have been helpful, though whether because of placebo or physiological action is unknown. Equally, there are anecdotal reports from patients that complementary treatments have not been helpful. Different professionals will come to different conclusions, but it seems prudent to conclude that there is no clear evidence for ruling out these methods nor for recommending them at the moment.

Complementary medical approaches take a holistic approach, and this holistic approach includes diet (particularly in Ayurvedic and Chinese medical traditions). Food can act as an asthma trigger, and food sensitivity may contribute to allergic processes. In fact, there is evidence, derived from conventional scientific methods, that dietary factors may be important in asthma: for example, that magnesium deficiency may be involved (Britton et al 1994, Carey et al 1996). A healthy diet including plenty of green vegetables (but avoiding oranges and citric fruits which contain a substance related to aspirin) may help. Some patients find avoidance of dairy, egg, or wheat products helpful, though all these dietary modifications are very patient specific – patients only benefit if the food acts a trigger (see section on food triggers, Ch. 3). Thus, the dietary component of complementary medicines may be consistent with conventional medicine in some cases.

Whatever the status of these complementary or dietary treatments, it is important that the patient should treat them as complementary rather than alternative. The difference between 'complementary' and 'alternative' is crucial from the point of view of safety of the patient. An alternative medicine is treated as a substitute for the conventional medicine. A complementary medicine is added on to the conventional medicine.

Patients who have strongly positive views about complementary medicines are unlikely to be convinced by a health professional telling them they are wrong. For example:

Box 6.10 A case of fatal attraction to attractive medicine

An example of the fatal alternative use of a non-conventional medicine is provided by an asthmatic woman in Devon who was sold a special new type of vitamin which she was told would cure her asthma. The woman stopped taking her conventional prophylactic treatment once she started the vitamins. She died from an asthma attack. For whatever reason, she was unable to talk to a health professional before starting on this course of action.

> *Nurse*: 'I can tell you that there is no proper scientific evidence supporting acupuncture. Frankly, I think you would be wasting your time and money.'
>
> *Patient*: (thinks) Well she would say that wouldn't she. Put her out of a job otherwise.

It is far better to act as missionaries do and incorporate the complementary medicine into a management plan which is open and accepted by all. A straight denial of the complementary medicine will merely serve to drive it underground, in the same way that illegal drugs are used despite being illegal. Patients will do what they want.

Complementary medicine can be introduced into the self-management plan in the sense of a steroid-sparing agent. However, when doing so there must be clear emphasis on assessment. So long as assessment is present, then the patient is not at risk. Once assessment is discontinued, then the patient will be at risk, as will be any patient whose anti-inflammatory medicine is insufficient. The following illustrates the kind of approach which might be taken

> 'Of course I am happy for you to try acupuncture. Actually I think it is a good idea.' *Note that confirming statements enhance liking and increase credibility.* 'Let's see whether it works. Keep going with your normal medicine for a few weeks – acupuncture takes a while to start working – and measure your peak flow. If acupuncture is working, your peak flow may improve. If your peak flow improves for a period of time, we could try decreasing your inhaled steroid. If the acupuncture is working then we should be able to decrease without any effect on your peak flow. You see, acupuncture works with some people and not others and we need to check it does actually work with you.' *In fact, if acupuncture does work, then it is highly likely it does not work effectively with all people. However, the last statement also provides a clear reason for assessment.*
>
> 'Acupuncture also works quite slowly, so we need to assess over a period of time. Come back and see me and we can measure how you are getting on. Let me know when you have started the acupuncture, and then we will make an appointment for review.'

In the illustration above, the health professional is managing the patient with a conventional trial of steroid reduction, but the trial of steroid reduction coincides with the introduction of acupuncture. Of course, using this method it is not possible to say whether the acupuncture is having an effect or whether natural variation in the disease would be responsible for reduced steroid need, but from a practical point of view it doesn't matter. The patient is being managed in a safe way. The patient still takes conventional anti-inflammatory medicine and is being assessed. The patient's beliefs are not being denied. The patient is open and honest with the health professional. The relationship between the health professional and patient is preserved.

COPING STRATEGIES

Coping refers to the patient's way of dealing with unpleasant events. The patient may *either* be aware of coping strategies, *or* only become aware when pointed out by someone else, *or* may not recognise the coping strategy at all. Leventhal, Diefenback & Leventhal (1992) suggests that when people cope with unpleasant events, they have two kinds of reaction: a rational cognitive reaction (the kind of reaction consistent with cost – benefit analysis) and an emotional or irrational reaction, where the patient is coping on an emotional level. It is this emotional form of reaction which is discussed in this section.

Self-perceptions

The label of asthma can affect self-concept, and can affect both the personal self and social self (Ch. 2). As a way of protecting the personal self, the patient may deny having asthma, and the consequences of denial have already been referred to in earlier sections. Nevertheless, it is important to note the motivational basis for this denial in some cases, as it can be very difficult to change.

In addition to the personal self, having asthma can affect the social self. The effect of asthma on the social self is particularly important for people for whom self-presentation is salient, for example amongst adolescents. Asthmatic teenagers and young adults are particularly at risk for asthma mortality when compared with asthmatics at other ages, and the impact of self-presentation may be one factor. In addition, the teenager may be in the process of rejecting parental influence, including parental influence in the management of asthma. Becoming independent from parents can, in some cases, involve becoming independent of the medicines that the parents have advocated for so long.

Dealing with young adults needs attention to their relationship with both parents and friends. In particular, it can be helpful to ensure that the teenager is treated like an adult rather than a child. However, it is also useful to discuss with patients how asthma impacts on their social self. For example, if the patient will not use an inhaler in public, then discussion in advance can help develop alternative coping strategies. For example, if the patient knows that he or she is about to go into a smoky situation, then it may be possible to go to the toilet and have a puff of a bronchodilator before entering the smoky situation, rather than find the need when there. Many young adults are concerned that having asthma should not label them as disabled or ill in any way, and a style of management which emphasises the normality of having asthma may help. Young people may be particularly sensitive to the styling of asthma devices. Devices that are compact and that can be used quickly and discretely when needed make public use easier. Fortunately, many manufacturers are now aware of this problem and are beginning to think about making devices of the future more acceptable as consumer objects.

Finally, although some asthmatics find asthma socially stigmatising, this is not invariably the case. I have come across adolescents who say that having asthma is actually a social asset because it provides a topic of conversation and interest which helps social integration. Negative self-perceptions depend not only on the patient but also on other people the patient knows and interacts with.

Problem- versus emotion-focused coping

Problem-focused coping occurs when the aim is to overcome or manage the problem in some way. Emotion-focused coping occurs when the aim is to reduce the negative emotions brought on by the problem (see Ch. 3). Both problem-focused and emotion-focused copers can be noncompliant, but they fail to comply for different reasons.

If problem-focused copers fail to comply with instructions, it is almost invariably because the patient has worked out a 'better' way of coping with the problem. In particular, patients who empower themselves more by adopting a more variable pattern of inhaled steroid use than recommended often do so because they believe that theirs is an effective strategy for taking the lowest amount of inhaled steroids needed. Perhaps such patients are correct. The issue really is not whether patients are behaving as instructed but whether the goals of asthma management are achieved: namely, safety from risk, good quality of life, and maintenance of body tissue. If patients who adopt a more variable pattern of medication use are free of exacerbations, if they have a frequency of bronchodilator use which is consistent with prophylactic medicine use (fewer bronchodilators than anti-inflammatories prescribed) then the patient's self-management plan is effective. Noncompliance is not a problem. On the other hand, if the patient's control is unsatisfactory in one way or another (e.g., needing courses of oral steroids and emergency treatment) then the variable pattern of anti-inflammatory medicine use *is* a problem and needs to be sorted out. Such patients respond to a rational approach where various options and outcomes are discussed. For example:

> *Nurse*: 'I see you have had four courses of oral steroids in the last year. How do you feel about this?'
>
> *Patient*: 'Well, obviously it is not very good.'
>
> *Nurse*: 'You actually have some more options open to you, you know. Shall I run through them?'
>
> *Patient*: 'Okay.'
>
> *Nurse*: 'Basically you have an option of a low regular dose of inhaled steroids and end up having lots of oral steroids; or you can have a higher dose of inhaled steroids and end up having less oral steroids. Actually, if you are worried about side effects, the second choice is much better for you.'

For problem-focused copers, it often helps to encourage them to work out a solution for themselves. Such patients are more likely to do something if they think they have decided it for themselves. Of course, not all problem-focused copers fail to comply. If the patient believes the practical solution to the problem of health care is to rely entirely on the health professional, then the result will be a highly compliant patient – though not one who will take appropriate action if instructions are not given exactly.

Noncompliance by emotion-focused copers is much more difficult to deal with. Emotion-focused copers often empower themselves less than recommended. The reason is that by exerting control over decisions, the emotion-focused coper is made more aware of asthma, and such awareness is avoided by people who cope by avoiding unpleasant emotions. In addition, emotion-focused copers are less likely to attend the asthma clinic, because the clinic itself elicits unhappy emotions in the patient. Emotion-focused copers can also overmedicate, because overmedication can be a strategy for avoiding the emotional impact of having to alter steroid dose. Attributing health outcomes to chance can also be a feature of the emotion-focused coper, since, in so doing, the patient is able to avoid the emotional impact of taking asthma-related care.

Although the management of emotion-focused copers is often going to be problematic, two strategies may help. If the patient is avoiding treatment and visits, the health professional should try to make the visit to the asthma clinic as pleasant as possible. Emotion-focused copers respond well to situations which provide positive feelings, so if the health professional makes a special effort to provide 'socio-emotional stroking' – in practice saying how wonderful the patient is – then the visit to the asthma clinic may turn out a pleasant experience after all. A second strategy is to avoid making the self-management plan too complex. Complexity and control add to the emotional salience of asthma, and a simple plan (with relatively few different types of medicine and which is comfortably high in anti-inflammatory medicine for the needs of the patient) may avoid exacerbations which arise because the patient fails to increase levels of medicine or to self-refer when needed.

Attention focus

When looking at a rose growing on a dung heap, do you notice the rose or the dung? The answer depends on attentional focus. Some people tend to notice the positive side of a situation and some the negative side. The idea of attentional focus also applies to asthma. If a patient only notices the good things in life, that patient may fail to notice asthma symptoms.

Although much noncompliance involves consistent under- or overmedication, another type of very important noncompliance occurs when the patient fails to increase medication or seek assistance when symptoms and PEF deteriorate. When asked, some patients will be perfectly aware of when and how to respond to worsening symptoms, but simply fail to do so in practice. Such patients respond to their asthma as though they simply don't notice it.

Failure to attend to asthma symptoms causes problems for asthma management, but, as a psychological coping strategy, repression of unpleasant emotional experiences is by no means unusual. Some people find that they can keep going only so long as they don't focus

Box 6.11 Brittle asthma

Brittle asthma refers to patients whose PEF suddenly falls quickly and without warning. Research by Professor Jon Ayres on brittle asthma shows that there are two types of brittle asthmatic who attend his brittle asthma clinic:

- patients whose PEF is typically stable but who suddenly have a catastrophic decline in lung function
- patients whose PEF starts to drop and they simply do not respond quickly enough or at all to the increase in symptoms and drop in PEF, *even though they have been told and know what to do.*

The former patients are physiologically brittle; they simply have sudden changes in physiological functioning. The latter patients are brittle for psychological reasons – their brittleness is associated with an inability to respond to worsening asthma. Many of the psychological brittles have a history of psychological problems, such as abuse as children.

Note: Brittle asthmatics should be referred to a specialist (see Ch. 5).

attention on the less pleasant aspects of life. Noticing the rose is a way of avoiding seeing the dung. It is unlikely, therefore, that a general style of coping with unpleasant emotional experiences will be easily changed.

Patients who fail to attend to their asthma are managed best by adopting a relatively simple self-management plan. The device and regimen should be convenient for the patient. The level of anti-inflammatory medicine needs to be sufficiently high on a regular basis to prevent frequent exacerbations which may not be responded to adequately. In addition, if patients still require emergency treatment, they should be advised to take a conservative course of action to ensure that as soon as they notice problems they obtain a high level of assistance – for example, going straight to accident and emergency rather than calling out the GP first.

Just as seeing the rose and not the dung limits the information available to a person, so seeing the dung and not the rose is also limiting. Another form of attentional focus is found in patients who become over-preoccupied with asthma. Over-preoccupation with asthma compromises quality of life rather than physiological risk.

Patients who are over-preoccupied with asthma may need specialist help to reduce asthma-specific anxiety. Treatment involves making the asthma more predictable, and using the increased predictability of asthma to focus on topics other than asthma. In summary, underattention to asthma symptoms leads to risk of exacerbations; overattention to asthma symptoms impairs quality of life.

NONCOMPLIANCE WITH BRONCHODILATORS

This chapter has focused on noncompliance with anti-inflammatory medicine, rather than with bronchodilators. Bronchodilators are prescribed on a PRN basis – the patient takes them when needed – so the criterion for compliance can not be defined in terms of doing other than instructed. However, bronchodilator use can be examined in terms of whether it is appropriate or not, that is, whether bronchodilators are being used at an appropriate level of PEF. Two studies where PEF values were compared with bronchodilator use came to somewhat similar conclusions (Kinsman, Dirks & Dahlem 1980, Mawhinney et al 1993): only about one third of patients were using their bronchodilator appropriately. The remainder divided into two groups of approximately equal size: about half underused their bronchodilators (i.e., failed to use it even when lung function was very poor), whereas the other half overused (i.e., used their bronchodilator when lung function was near normal).

Of course, symptoms and lung function are poorly related in some patients, and bronchodilator use is strongly associated with symptoms. Thus, some of the inappropriate use may arise from the inconsistent relationship between symptoms and PEF. Patients respond to symptoms, not to PEF. However, the researchers also found personality correlates with under- or overuse. Overusers tend to be more anxious generally than underusers. Underusers had greater confidence in their ability to deal with asthma. In fact, there is a general trend for highly anxious patients to take their anti-inflammatory medicine regularly, and overuse on bronchodilators. By contrast, low-anxiety patients are less likely to take their anti-inflammatory medicines, but they underuse on bronchodilators – so that when PEF drops as a result of inadequate anti-inflammatory medicine, they fail to compensate with bronchodilators. The relationship between noncompliance in anti-inflammatory and bronchodilator medicines is important because it is not always possible to detect underuse of anti-inflammatory drugs through an increased use of bronchodilator.

CONCLUSIONS

One of the conclusions to be drawn about noncompliance is that there is no such thing as 'the noncompliant patient'. The expression 'noncompliant patient' implies that there is a single type of patient who can be managed in one particular way. Quite the reverse is true: there are many different behaviours which can be labelled non-compliant; these behaviours occur for many different reasons; and the behaviours have many different outcomes on quality of life and risk. Management of noncompliance requires the health professional to focus on the individual characteristics of the patient, in terms of behaviour, motivation and outcome.

REFERENCES

Ayres J G 1986 Acute asthma in Asian patients: hospital admissions and duration of stay in a district with a high immigrant population. British Journal of Diseases of the Chest 80: 242–248

Bender B, Milgrom H 1996 Compliance with asthma therapy: a case for shared responsibility. Journal of Asthma 33: 199–202

Bhopal R S 1986 The inter-relationship of folk, traditional and western medicine with an Asian Community in Britain. Social Science and Medicine 22: 99–105

Blessing-Moore J 1996 Does asthma education change behavior? To know is not to do. Chest 109: 9–11

Bosley C M, Parry D T, Cochrane G M 1994 Patient compliance with inhaled medication: does combined beta agonists with corticosteroids improve compliance? European Respiratory Journal 7: 504–509

Britton J, Pavord I, Richards K et al 1994 Dietary magnesium, lung function, wheezing, and airway hyperreactivity in a random adult population sample. Lancet 344: 357–362

Carey O J, Cookson J B, Britton J, Tattersfield A E 1996 The effect of lifestyle on wheeze, atopy, and bronchial hyper-reactivity in Asian and White children. American Journal of Respiratory Critical Care Medicine 153: 537–540

Chemlik F, Doughty A 1994 Objective measurements of compliance in asthma treatment. Annals of Allergy 73: 527–532

Cramer J A, Mattson R H, Prevey M L, Scheyer R D, Ouellette V L 1989 How often is medication taken as prescribed? A novel assessment technique. Journal of the American Medical Association 261: 3273–3277

Crompton G K 1988 New inhalation devices. European Respiratory Journal 1: 679–680

Dompeling E, van Grunsven P M, van Schayck C P, Folgering H, Molema J, van Weel C 1992 Treatment with inhaled steroids in asthma and chronic bronchitis: long-term compliance and inhaler technique. Family Practice 9: 161–166

Fisher E B, Sussman L K, Arfken C, Harrison D, Munro J, Sykes R K, Sylvia S, Strunk R C 1994 Targeting high risk groups. Chest 106 (suppl.): S248–259

Horn C R, Clark T J H, Cochrane G M 1990 Compliance with inhaled therapy and morbidity from asthma. Respiratory Medicine 84: 67–70

Hyland M E, Ley A, Fisher D W, Woodward V 1995 Measurement of psychological distress in asthma management programs. British Journal of Clinical Psychology 34: 601–611

Kinsman R A, Dirks J F, Dahlem N W 1980 Noncompliance to prescribed as needed (PRN) medication use in asthma: usage patterns and patient characteristics. Journal of Psychosomatic Research 24: 97–107

Leventhal H, Diefenback M, Leventhal E A 1992 Illness cognition: using common sense to understand treatment adherence and affect cognition interactions. Cognitive Therapy and Research 16: 143–163

Mawhinney H, Spector S L, Heitjan D, Kinsman R A, Dirks J F, Pines I 1993 As-needed medication use in asthma: usage patterns and patient characteristics. Journal of Asthma 30: 61–71

Omerod L P 1995 Asian acute asthma readmission reassessed: Blackburn 1991–1992. Respiratory Medicine 89: 415–417

Rosenstock I M (1974) The health belief model and preventive health behavior. Health Education Monographs 2: 328–335

Royal Pharmaceutical Society 1996 Partnership in medicine taking: a consultative document. Royal Pharmaceutical Society, London

Strunk R C, Mrazek D A, Furman G S W, Barecque J F 1985 Psychological and physiological characteristics associated with death due to asthma in childhood: a case controlled study. Journal of the American Medical Association 254: 1193–1198

Policy decisions and organisational matters

7

CONTENTS

Asthma clinics can be organised and run in several different ways. The organisation of an asthma clinic reflects policy decisions which are taken on the way asthma care should be delivered. Different practices may have different policies. This chapter describes issues and options available in organising an asthma clinic.

PRACTICE PROTOCOL

Practices should have their own protocol which describes how asthma is managed in the practice. The protocol should cover issues such as:

- objective of the asthma clinic
- method of referral to the clinic
- management structure of the clinic
- time allowed, time of day
- method of registration, recall policy and follow up
- information collected

- activities to be carried out during the running of the clinic
- prescription policy.

The purpose of a practice protocol is to provide a record of agreement between the members of the health care team about the way asthma is managed. It is important to ensure that all members of a team agree the protocol, and in large practices it can be an advantage for all the doctors and respiratory nurses to sign the protocol. In addition, the protocol provides protection for the practice nurse, particularly if the nurse writes prescriptions which are then signed by the doctor. If that is the procedure then it is important that there is a written record confirmed by the GP.

The protocol should change with changes in practice policy and should be agreed (perhaps by signature) by all members of the team.

AUDIT AND RECORD KEEPING

Audit and record keeping sound terribly dry and uninteresting, but really they are very important. One way of thinking about record keeping is as a kind of safety net. Careful records can prevent accidents from happening, in particular the inappropriate use of asthma medicines.

A limited amount of information should be recorded for each patient, and checked periodically as part of good clinical practice. Information which helps in maintaining a safety net includes that on drug prescription and emergency care provided. Information which helps in patient management includes a record of communication. Computers provide the ideal method for checking 'safety net' information, but this is perfectly possible using paper and pencil records.

Drug prescriptions

A record should be kept to show the number of asthma drug prescriptions in quarterly or half yearly periods (or on some other basis) for each patient. The record could be collected on a computer spreadsheet or by paper and pencil, and the exact type of information to be collected should be decided by the practice. Figure 7.1 provides an example of a paper and pencil version, where the patient's prescriptions in a period are simply added as a '1' each time the

Patient's name	Jan–Mar 1997	Apr–Jun 1997	Jul–Sep 1997	Oct–Dec 1997
Mrs Adam	Preventer: 1111 Reliever: 11	Preventer: 111 Reliever: 111	Preventer: 1111 Reliever: 11	
Mr Brown	Preventer: 11 Reliever: 11	Preventer: 1 Reliever: 111	Preventer: Reliever: 1111	

Fig. 7.1 Example of a prescription record.

prescription is given (equivalent versions can be computer presented). In this version, drugs are simply classified as 'preventer' and 'reliever', but a more complex form of counting is possible if preferred.

Figure 7.1 shows at a glance that Mrs Adam is managing reasonably well, but Mr Brown is taking fewer preventers than appropriate. The purpose of a prescription chart is to make the detection of irregularities easy. Some clinic computer programs have a warning which flashes up if the patient is taking an inappropriate ratio of bronchodilators to anti-inflammatory drugs, and such warnings provide an additional safety measure. Humans can make errors when scanning down a chart for information; computers do not – at least when they are working!

Note that this audit only provides a record of prescriptions, not what patients have actually taken (see Ch. 6). It may be that the ratio of preventers to relievers seems acceptable but in reality the patient is only obtaining or using relievers. It is therefore a good idea to make a note against high bronchodilator use irrespective of the

Box 7.1 Prescription records and litigation

Litigation is becoming increasingly common in medicine. It might be possible to argue that a practice was negligent if large numbers of bronchodilators were being prescribed by repeat prescription without checking.

number of steroids inhalers, particularly in relation to emergency care provision.

Emergency care provision

Emergency care provision should be recorded, but it is useful to know about emergency care under different headings. One possibility is to use the following six headings: hospital inpatient, Accident and Emergency, nebulisations, out of hours call-out by GP, unscheduled clinic visit, and courses of oral steroids. Record keeping can be achieved either on a computer record or by using paper and pencil chart, and the time scale should be in 6-monthly or yearly periods. (see Fig. 7.2) Such a record is particularly useful on routine review, but also to indicate whether the frequency of review needs to be increased. If emergency care provision is recorded on a chart for the practice as a whole – rather than kept only in the patient's notes – then the standard for the practice will be apparent. This figure can then be used as an audit of one aspect of the quality of care provided.

If for any individual patient, there are high levels of emergency care, then the patient's prescription record (Fig. 7.1) should be

Patient's name	1995	1996	1997	1998
Mrs Adam	Admission A & E Nebulisations Unscheduled visits Oral steroids: 1	Admission A & E Nebulisations Unscheduled visits: 1 Oral steroids		
Mr Brown	Admission A & E: 1 Nebulisations Unscheduled visits: 111 Oral steroids: 11	Admission: 11 A & E: 1 Nebulisations Unscheduled visits Oral steroids: 11		

Fig. 7.2 The record shows at a glance that Mr Brown is having many problems.

examined. High levels of emergency care may result from very severe asthma, or may result from inadequate anti-inflammatory medication. In either case, review is needed, possibly with referral. The record of emergency care provision is therefore helpful for individual patient management. The information contained in Figures 7.1 and 7.2 quickly shows that Mr Brown's management may be unsatisfactory.

Information about drug use and emergency treatment, when reviewed regularly, provides a useful safety net. In addition, when summarised for the practice as a whole, such information allows assessment of the effectiveness of asthma management. For example, high levels of prescribed short-acting β-agonists (i.e., many more bronchodilators than anti-inflammatories) would indicate that the BTS guidelines are not being adhered to.

Consultations record

A record of consultations – what is said to the patient and what the patient says – should be kept in some form, and the record should include a comment about how the patient is responding to asthma. Consultation records should be retained on a patient-by-patient basis (e.g., attached to notes). The particular form and complexity of the record will vary between practices but should not be so simple that it includes only two boxes to tick: compliant and noncompliant! Consultation records are useful to check that appropriate information has been provided to the patient. For example, the record can show whether or not the patient has received a particular information leaflet – it is easy to miss out on information in isolated cases if a record is not kept. An easy form of a communication record is to keep it as a checklist, with a space for comments, and an example is shown in Figure 7.3

Other audit records

The percentage of patients with a diagnosis of asthma provides an estimate of the diagnostic accuracy of the practice. Assuming that the national average is in the order of 4–5% of patients with asthma, any figure widely different would suggest that there may be problems with diagnosis. For example, if only 2% of the adult practice population are diagnosed as asthmatic, then there is likely to be a problem of diagnosis.

Topics are ticked as appropriate

Patient: ....

	Visit date: 10th March	Visit date: 20th October	Visit date: 2nd May	Visit date:	Visit date:
Nature of asthma	X	X	X		
Drug action	X	X			
Technique	X	X	X		
Symptoms	X	X	X		
PEF		X	X		
Bothers			X		
Time off work/ school		X	X		
Comments			Poor co-ordination		

Fig. 7.3 Example of a consultations record.

CLINIC APPOINTMENTS AND REPEAT PRESCRIPTIONS

Length and time of visit

How long should the clinic appointment be? Should the length of the appointment be variable for different people. Should patients know how long the appointment is for? The answer to each of these questions reflects a policy decision about clinic appointments. Let us consider the question of variability of appointment times first. It is always difficult to predict how long a patient will need, but nevertheless, newly diagnosed patients who require education will, on average, need more time than 'old lags' who are visiting for the purpose of monitoring and review. It may be useful to organise asthma clinics using a time frame where the purpose of the visit is identified in advance. Of course, if prediction is difficult or is often wrong then the system breaks down, so this is not a recommendation for all practices.

The average length of time for visits varies considerably between different practices (with a minimum of about 15 min, 20–30 min being common, but longer times also being used). Longer is not necessarily better. The aim is to achieve effective use of time rather than just use time. Nevertheless, at early stages of treatment, patients may need up to 45 min.

Some clinics may opt not to have formal clinic 'sessions' but to run an opportunistic drop-in service. Some patients prefer the drop-in service, whereas others prefer appointment visits. Equally, some patients find day-time visits difficult (e.g., because they are working), whereas others find evening visits difficult (e.g., because they are looking after children). Although no arrangement will suit everyone, convenience to the patient should be one factor to take into account, as convenience may have a substantial effect on compliance.

Information booklets and telephones

Time may be saved in two ways. First, by providing patients with information booklets. Information booklets are not as effective as individual discussion with patients, but they are better than nothing and can be useful as an adjunct to discussion. In selecting an information booklet, the health professional should consider that, of the several kinds of booklet available, some may suit some patients more than others. It is not a matter of selecting 'the best available', because there is no such thing. What is 'best' depends on the patient.

A second strategy for time saving is to use the telephone. Although not all patients have telephones, it is possible to instigate a policy of review by telephone. Once the health professional has established a relationship with the patient, then monitoring clinic visits can be carried out over the telephone in some cases. The use of the telephone may be preferred by some patients because of reduced travelling time. The telephone is useful in monitoring factual information (e.g., frequency of symptoms or frequency of reliever medicines used), but not always effective at monitoring emotional information.

Repeat prescriptions

How many months should elapse before repeat visits? How many repeat prescriptions should a patient have before review – or should review be based on time interval alone? Should restriction of repeat prescriptions be used as a way of forcing patients to come to the clinic or just to turn up to the surgery? Note that if it is difficult to obtain a prescription, then patients may simply fail to do so, leading to increased risk, which surely is not the purpose of the policy – whom are the clinics for? Should a repeat prescription policy be the same for all patients, or should patients be put into different categories whereby some need less surveillance than others?

Apart from following the requirements for reimbursement – which is that patients should be seen at least once per year – practices operate on a variety of policies, though there is little evidence to support one course of action over another. In addition, what may work for one practice may not work for another. The advantage of uniformity in approach to repeat prescriptions (i.e., having the same policy for all patients) is that it is easier to justify to patients, and is also easier to administer – patients do talk to each other and it is always easy to blame 'the system' which requires attendance rather than allowing attendance to be optional. The disadvantage of uniformity is that patients are likely to have different needs or competencies with regard to repeat prescriptions, and for some patients the additional visiting is unnecessary – and unpopular with patients.

Some patients are highly reluctant to attend the clinic. Whether withdrawal of drugs should be used as a way of ensuring clinic attendance is open to dispute. On the positive side, such measures do at least ensure patient attendance; on the negative side, there is always the risk that drugs will be underused as a way of reducing the need for visits.

Gatekeeping

Who determines whether the patient can see the respiratory nurse if the patient wants to? Does the same receptionist make appointments for the doctor and for the respiratory nurse? What training has the receptionist been given specifically with regard to asthma? These questions relate to a problem which emerges from time to time in large practices: sometimes the nurses do not feel that the urgency of asthma care is sufficiently appreciated by the receptionist. Broadly speaking, asthma visits can be divided into two kinds: visits for which there is no time urgency, and visits for which there is time urgency. The respiratory nurse will know at once what category a visit comes under, but a receptionist may not. The solution is training for the receptionist (and in large practices, this may mean having a specialist nurse receptionist) and including the receptionist in the formulation of the practice protocol.

TARGETED OR NONTARGETED MANAGEMENT?

Should all patients receive the same amount of time or should the health professional's time be directed to those who need it most? The answer to this question depends to some extent on resourcing and to some extent on beliefs about equity. It is more equitable to make the same amount of time available to all patients, but there may not be the resources to do so. In addition, some patients may want more support than others, and, in any case, the impact of asthma is not equivalent across different patients. Thus, there are both financial and ethical reasons why a policy may be taken to target resources. The downside of targeting, however, is that there will always be the odd person in the nontargeted group who actually needs the level of help of those in the targeted group. A natural consequence of targeting is that you will not get it right every time.

If the decision is to target resources, then one strategy is to target those patients who are most at risk of acute exacerbations. There are many factors which increase the risk of acute exacerbations and which have been discussed in previous chapters, but three which are particularly relevant to policy decisions are:

- severity
- social class
- family dysfunction.

Severity

Severity of asthma increases asthma risk. One policy decision may be to review the more severe asthmatics (in particular, Steps 4 and 5) more frequently. That is, the more severe patients have a shorter period between clinic visits than less severe patients. A suggestion made in Chapter 4 was that patients should be involved in deciding the time interval between clinic visits. Although this remains a good idea, patients respond well to information about 'what is normal', so their preference can be solicited in terms of an increase or decrease in relation to 'what is normal'. One possible approach for targeting is to describe 'what is normal' differently for patients of different severity.

Social class and ethnic background

Lower economic status and social class are both associated with poorer asthma control, including mortality (Higgins & Britton 1995). In one study, 19% of asthma attendances at Accident and Emergency departments were from patients who were unemployed, compared with the then national average of 8% (Partridge, Latouche & Thurston 1997). Of course, there are several reasons why patients from poorer backgrounds may choose asthma care at the A & E department, but these statistics are coupled with many others which show that, overall, the management of patients from lower social class background is less satisfactory. Higher than average A & E care is also needed by people from ethnic minority backgrounds (Ormerod 1995). One possible policy decision, therefore, would be to target resources more to those who are from more economically deprived or minority ethnic backgrounds – the two are sometimes associated.

Family dysfunction

Family dysfunction and emotional reactions from other members of the family lead to greater need for emergency asthma care (Wamboldt et al 1995). Although the health professional is unlikely to make much impact on dysfunctional family relations, awareness that family problems impact on asthma management may be useful in managing such patients. In particular, it may be necessary to discuss with the patient not only the patient's response to asthma but also the response of other family members.

Type of practice

Practices have different records of asthma care. 'Asthma interested' practices tend to have higher asthma drug-prescribing costs but lower costs of antibiotics. In addition, the practice attended by the patient affects the level of risk of having to attend Accident and

Emergency for asthma treatment. Data from one study (Griffiths et al 1997) showed that single-handed practices and those that had high night-visiting rates resulted in a greater need for hospital emergency care in their asthmatic patients. It would not seem unreasonable if tired, overstretched staff provided less effective care. The management and motivation of staff is therefore important in the organisation of asthma care.

DRUG RATIONING

Recently developed asthma drugs are more expensive than older ones. New devices can also be more expensive than older ones. In the case of older drugs, generic manufacturers usually sell at a lower price than the original patent holder. However, many generic drugs are now available in the newer, more expensive type of inhalers. Not only are asthma drugs expensive, but also health care budgets, including prescribing budgets, are limited. These are uncomfortable facts of life.

The general policy of the NHS is to obtain the best value for money available, and this means that some forms of treatment are rationed. Rationing already takes a variety of forms in the NHS. For example, treatments such as fertility treatment may be rationed by the number of tries allowed, others are rationed by the length of waiting list, and others are simply unavailable. At the time of writing, portable liquid oxygen is not available on the NHS, though this is likely to change. Health rationing is an emotive issue and one with which many health professionals feel uncomfortable. Nevertheless, health rationing is in itself not new. What is new is rationing on the basis of cost. Other forms of rationing – triage in the case of accidents, and prioritisation for transplant organs – have featured in health care for many years.

With regard to asthma the NHS policy is to obtain effective treatment at minimum cost. Consequently, generic medicines are recommended, as these are cheaper. The ethical arguments are not entirely one sided. Pharmaceutical or device manufacturers of branded products argue that the cost is needed to pay for the development of new drugs and devices, and that they put some of their profit into education and other support for asthma. The NHS response is that impoverished pharmaceutical companies are rare.

Irrespective of these arguments, the internal economy of the NHS has led general practices to be much more conscious of the cost of drugs, including the cost of asthma drugs.

Pharmaceutical companies are unlikely to invest in the considerable cost (about £200 million) of launching a new drug if the new drug is not, in some way, an improvement on the old. Although device development can be cheaper than drug development, it normally happens that new devices are better than ones which have been developed before. Hence, it seems entirely plausible that new and more expensive drugs and devices can enhance quality of life – either through better asthma control or through improved safety. Whether the improvement in quality of life can be justified by the cost is a different matter, and decisions to prescribe drugs are not entirely independent of economic concepts such as 'value for money' and 'total drug budget'. Thus, the choice of drugs – for example, whether to introduce a long-acting β-agonist or to increase steroid dose at Step 3 can be influenced by the relative cost of these two alternatives, and not just the quality-of-life gain involved.

General practices often have patterns of prescribing which reflect implicit or explicit decisions about which drugs (or which manufacturers' drugs) should be used, and where the decision to prescribe is based not only on efficacy but also cost. There is considerable variation in prescribing policy. Asthma care often involves team work among a group of health professionals, and because emotive issues easily get swept under the carpet, it is best to make asthma rationing decisions explicit to all members of the team. In particular, it is helpful to make the values on which the rationing decisions are made, if they are made, known to all health professionals concerned.

CONCLUSIONS

Organisational decisions need to be made in delivering asthma care in a primary care setting. Different policies may suit different practices, but a clear setting out and discussion of policy will be helpful for all members of the primary health care team.

REFERENCES

Griffiths C J, Sturdy P, Naish J et al 1997 Hospital admissions for asthma in east London: associations with characteristics of local general practices, prescribing and population. British Medical Journal 314: 482–486
Higgins B G, Britton J R 1995 Geographical and social class effects on asthma mortality in England and Wales. Respiratory Medicine 89: 341–346
Ormerod L P 1995 Asian acute asthma readmission reassessed: Blackburn 1991–1992. Respiratory Medicine 89: 415–417
Partridge M, Latouche D, Thurston J G 1997 A national census of those attending Accident and Emergency departments with asthma. Journal of Accident and Emergency Medicine 14: 16–20
Wamboldt F, Wamboldt M X, Gavin L A et al 1995 Parental criticism and treatment outcome in adolescents hospitalised for severe chronic asthma. Journal of Psychosomatic Research 39: 995–1005

Appendix 1: Asthma Bother Profile

- Asthma affects people in many different ways
- For some people asthma causes very little bother
- For others, asthma is very troublesome
- The purpose of this questionnaire is to find out **how much your asthma bothers you overall**

PART ONE

Would you please provide the following information before going on to the rest of the questionnaire:

Age ____ **Male** ◯ **Female** ◯ Please tick ✓

Please tick ✓ **any** month when your asthma bothers you

Jan ◯ Feb ◯ Mar ◯ Apr ◯ May ◯ Jun ◯

Jul ◯ Aug ◯ Sep ◯ Oct ◯ Nov ◯ Dec ◯

If you have had asthma for less than 12 months, please state for many months you have had it ________

(Please write the number of months on the line)

Please write todays date here: ____________________

PART TWO

Please answer the following questions by putting a tick next to reply which **most closely applies to you** ✓

Please don't spend too long thinking about each question. It is your **general impression** which is important.

How much does your asthma bother you at your **paid work?**

- ◯ No bother at all
- ◯ Minor irritation
- ◯ Slight bother
- ◯ Moderate bother
- ◯ A lot of bother
- ◯ Makes my life a misery

Tick here if unemployed or retired **because of asthma** ◯

Tick here if retired ◯

Please tick one only ✓

Overall, how much does your asthma bother you when you do **jobs around the house?**

- ◯ No bother at all
- ◯ Minor irritation
- ◯ Slight bother
- ◯ Moderate bother
- ◯ A lot of bother
- ◯ Makes my life a misery
- ◯ None of these really apply to me

Such as:
housework
shopping
home maintenance
gardening
child care

Please tick one only ✓

Overall, how much does your asthma bother your **social life?** Such as: visiting friends walking with friends talking with friends going to pubs/restaurants parties	◯ No bother at all ◯ Minor irritation ◯ Slight bother ◯ Moderate bother ◯ A lot of bother ◯ Makes my life a misery Please tick one only ✓
Overall, how much does your asthma bother your **personal life?** Such as: love life personal relationships family life	◯ No bother at all ◯ Minor irritation ◯ Slight bother ◯ Moderate bother ◯ A lot of bother ◯ Makes my life a misery ◯ None of these really apply to me Please tick one only ✓
If involved in **leisure activities,** how much does your asthma bother you? Such as: walking for pleasure, sports, exercise, travelling, holidays **As well as** ticking one of the replies opposite, please tick here **if** you **can't do** some of these sorts of things **because of asthma**	◯ No bother at all ◯ Minor irritation ◯ Slight bother ◯ Moderate bother ◯ A lot of bother ◯ Makes my life a misery ◯ Don't want to do these sorts of things anyway Please tick one only ✓

PART THREE

Here are some things which often happen to people when they have asthma.

How much is each a bother to you?

How much does your asthma bother you when you **sleep?**

- ◯ No bother at all
- ◯ Minor irritation
- ◯ Slight bother
- ◯ Moderate bother
- ◯ A lot of bother
- ◯ Makes my life a misery

Such as:
coughing at night
waking at night
waking early

Please tick one only ✓

How much does the **cost** of your **asthma medicines** bother you?

- ◯ No bother at all
- ◯ Minor irritation
- ◯ Slight bother
- ◯ Moderate bother
- ◯ A lot of bother
- ◯ Makes my life a misery

As well as ticking one of the replies opposite, please tick here **if** you get **free prescriptions** ◯

Please tick one only ✓

How much does the **inconvenience** or **embarassment** of **taking your asthma medicines** bother you?

- No bother at all
- Minor irritation
- Slight bother
- Moderate bother
- A lot of bother
- Makes my life a misery

Please tick one only ✓

How much do **coughs and colds** bother you?

- No bother at all
- Minor irritation
- Slight bother
- Moderate bother
- A lot of bother
- Makes my life a misery
- Never get coughs or colds

Please tick one only ✓

Feeling upset is also a bother. If your asthma makes you feel **anxious, depressed, tired** or **helpless**, how much does this bother you?

- No bother at all
- Minor irritation
- Slight bother
- Moderate bother
- A lot of bother
- Makes my life a misery
- My asthma never makes me feel this way

Please tick one only ✓

PART FOUR

Worries can also be a bother, particularly if you spend a lot of time worrying.

How much bother is the worry that you will have an **asthma attack** when visiting a **new place?**

- ◯ I never have this worry
- ◯ Minor irritation
- ◯ Slight bother
- ◯ Moderate bother
- ◯ A lot of bother
- ◯ Makes my life a misery

Please tick one only ✓

How much bother is the worry that you will catch a **cold**?

- ◯ I never have this worry
- ◯ Minor irritation
- ◯ Slight bother
- ◯ Moderate bother
- ◯ A lot of bother
- ◯ Makes my life a misery

Please tick one only ✓

How much bother is the worry that you will let others down?

Such as:
missed appointments
being off work
change of plans

- ◯ I never have this worry
- ◯ Minor irritation
- ◯ Slight bother
- ◯ Moderate bother
- ◯ A lot of bother
- ◯ Makes my life a misery

Please tick one only ✓

How much bother is the worry that **your health may get worse in the future?**

Such as:
increasing breathlessness
effects of medicines
being able to do less

- ◯ I never have this worry
- ◯ Minor irritation
- ◯ Slight bother
- ◯ Moderate bother
- ◯ A lot of bother
- ◯ Makes my life a misery

Please tick one only ✓

How much bother is the worry that you won't be able to cope with an **asthma attack?**

- ◯ I never have this worry
- ◯ Minor irritation
- ◯ Slight bother
- ◯ Moderate bother
- ◯ A lot of bother
- ◯ Makes my life a misery

Please tick one only ✓

PART FIVE

The purpose of this section is to find out what you think about the care and support you receive from the doctor's surgery.

For each of the following statements, please use a tick as before, to show overall – how true or untrue each statement is for you.

If my asthma was a problem, my doctor would see me quickly

- ◯ Very untrue
- ◯ Moderately untrue
- ◯ Slightly untrue
- ◯ Slightly true
- ◯ Moderately true
- ◯ Very true

Please tick one only ✓

I have confidence in my ability to deal with an asthma attack

- ◯ Very untrue
- ◯ Moderately untrue
- ◯ Slightly untrue
- ◯ Slightly true
- ◯ Moderately true
- ◯ Very true

Please tick one only ✓

I am sure about how my medicine works

- ◯ Very untrue
- ◯ Moderately untrue
- ◯ Slightly untrue
- ◯ Slightly true
- ◯ Moderately true
- ◯ Very true

Please tick one only ✓

Please turn over

My doctor/nurse has carefully explained how I should manage my asthma	◯ Very untrue ◯ Moderately untrue ◯ Slightly untrue ◯ Slightly true ◯ Moderately true ◯ Very true Please tick one only ✓
I think I am given the best care possible for my asthma	◯ Very untrue ◯ Moderately untrue ◯ Slightly untrue ◯ Slightly true ◯ Moderately true ◯ Very true Please tick one only ✓
I would like more general information about asthma	◯ Very untrue ◯ Moderately untrue ◯ Slightly untrue ◯ Slightly true ◯ Moderately true ◯ Very true Please tick one only ✓
I don't know when to call the doctor for my asthma	◯ Very untrue ◯ Moderately untrue ◯ Slightly untrue ◯ Slightly true ◯ Moderately true ◯ Very true Please tick one only ✓

Please tick here if you have attended the asthma clinic ◯

About how many times have you attended? ____________

Index

References to boxed material appear in italics.

About the PROFESSIONAL DEVELOPMENT RECORD

The United Kingdom Central Council (UKCC) PREP regulations require you to maintain a personal professional portfolio, in which you record evidence of your professional development.

This book provides you with excellent educational material to assist your study and develop your practice. Reading all or parts of it can contribute to your professional development.

The *Professional Development Record* (overleaf) is designed to help you record your study activity in your portfolio and show how it has enhanced your practice. To use the Record, you can do either of the following:

- photocopy the Record and place it directly into your portfolio, or
- use it as a basis for your own individual entry.

The aim of the Record is to help you plan how this book assists your professional development, to the benefit of yourself, your colleagues and your patients/clients.

Further information:

- If you do not have a portfolio and would like to purchase one, please contact your local bookseller or, in case of difficulty, phone our Customer Services Department on 0181 300 3322.
- If you need further information about PREP, you should contact the UKCC on: 0171 333 6550.

PROFESSIONAL DEVELOPMENT RECORD

Book (fill in author, title, year of publication, publisher):

Date of completion of book (or selections from book):

Duration of study time:

Reason for reading the book:

Intended learning outcomes:

Evaluation of material read:

Planned influence on practice:

Evaluation of influence on practice:

Learning outcomes achieved:

WITHDRAWN
from
STIRLING UNIVERSITY LIBRARY

33100128